Radiographic Examination in Blunt Abdominal Trauma

JAMES J. McCORT, M.D.

Director of Radiology, Santa Clara County Hospital,
San Jose, California;
Clinical Associate Professor of Radiology, Stanford University
Medical School, Palo Alto, California

W. B. SAUNDERS COMPANY
Philadelphia and London, 1966

W. B. Saunders Company: West Washington Square
                           Philadelphia, Pa. 19105

                           12 Dyott Street
                           London W. C. 1

Radiographic Examination in Blunt Abdominal Trauma

"Our study is man, as the subject of accidents or diseases."
OSLER

ACKNOWLEDGMENTS

The following colleagues have given me the opportunity of studying their patients and films: Herbert Abrams, Robert Allansmith, Joseph Brozda, Justin Colburn, Thomas N. Foster, T. Hattori, George Hoeffler, George Jacobson, Robert Jamplis, Howard Jones, George Magid, William Marshall, Tord Olin, Leo Rigler, John Rodenbaugh, Stanford Rossiter, Robert Ruskin, Eugene Saenger, Stefan Schatzki, William Thompson, John von Saltza, C. C. Wang, Lee Watanabe. Their help is gratefully acknowledged.

Mrs. Rosalie Foster and Miss Maxine Jordan are responsible for the drawings. Mr. Charles Taddo and his staff supplied the photographic reproductions.

Many valuable ideas were contributed by my associates: Virginia Raphael, George Easter, William McLaughlin and James Vaudagna.

Excellent articles on blunt abdominal trauma have appeared in recent years. The ideas of others have been freely utilized in assembling this material and the attempt has been made to give each author credit in the text. If, through oversight, proper credit has not been given to a writer, the author apologizes.

To paraphrase Sir William Osler, the physician who teaches is in turn taught by assistants and students. For years, the interns and residents on the Emergency Service of the Santa Clara County Hospital have prodded the author with questions about their patients. From this experience he was led to believe that this book might serve a useful purpose.

Contents

1

INTRODUCTION

Each year greater numbers of patients with closed abdominal trauma are seen in hospital emergency rooms. This is largely a result of the wider use of high speed vehicles and increased industrialization. According to the National Safety Council[1] accidents, including those due to motor vehicles, rank fourth as a cause of death in the United States.

Whether the patient survives his injury and to what extent complications develop depend on the adequacy of the immediate medical treatment.[3] A crucial factor in the success of treatment is the experience and judgment of the emergency room physician, who must be thoroughly trained in the care of accident victims. He functions most efficiently when backed by a team of consultants. A key member of the team is the radiologist.

Proper treatment of abdominal injury depends on prompt and accurate diagnosis. A correct evaluation of the type and extent of the patient's injuries must be made quickly and with the least possible manipulation of the accident victim. Van Wagoner[2] made an analysis of the records of 606 healthy adult males who were injured and who died in a hospital within two weeks of their admission. In one out of three patients in whom the main cause of death was abdominal trauma, the diagnosis was not made ante mortem.

With post-traumatic deformity of an extremity the need for radiographic examination is clear. Equally clear should be the need for radiography of the abdomen in the presence of contusions of the abdominal wall, fractures of the lower ribs and pelvis, or an unexplained fall in the hematocrit.

The value of the radiographic study is directly proportional to the interest and skill of the radiologist. It is most satisfactory when he personally supervises the examination. By using special diagnostic procedures, he can improve the accuracy of the study.

The author's cases were obtained mainly from the emergency service of the Santa Clara County Hospital and Medical Center. A number of interesting examples of abdominal trauma have been kindly provided by radiologic and surgical colleagues. Where these have been used, credit is given in the footnote. Because cases selected in this manner are not a random sample, statistical assessment of the reliability and frequency of occurrence of roentgen signs in abdominal trauma is not possible. In all cases used as illustrations, the diagnoses were confirmed at operation or autopsy unless otherwise noted.

In presenting the subject of blunt trauma to the abdomen, it is convenient to separate the injuries according to the organ system involved. Further subdivision (based on radiographic criteria) is made according to the severity and nature of the injury to each organ. In clinical practice multiple injuries are common.

Step by step analysis is required. The radiologist looks for signs of injury to the bones, muscles and fat. Then he attempts to determine whether the continuity of the organ is disturbed. Finally he searches for evidence of bleeding and the leakage of urine or intestinal contents into the peritoneal and retroperitoneal tissues.

This book is intended for the radiologist who is called to assist in the care of patients injured by blunt abdominal trauma. It is hoped that it will serve as a useful reference for all physicians who treat patients in the emergency room.

REFERENCES

1. Accident Facts. The National Safety Council, 425 N. Michigan Ave., Chicago, Ill. 60611, 1964.
2. Van Wagoner, F. H.: Died in hospital. A three year study of deaths following trauma. J. Trauma, 1:401-408, 1961.
3. Waller, J. A., Curran, R., and Noyes, F.: Traffic deaths. A preliminary study of urban and rural fatalities in California. California Med., 101:272-276, 1964.

ADDITIONAL REFERENCES

Braunstein, P. M., Moore, J. O., and Wade, P. A.: Preliminary findings of the effect of automotive safety design on injury patterns. Surg. Gynec. Obstet., 105:257-263, 1957.
Fitzgerald, J. B., Crawford, E. S., and DeBakey, M.: Surgical considerations of non-penetrating abdominal injuries: An analysis of 200 cases. Amer. J. Surg. 100:22-29, 1960.
Garrett, J. W., and Braunstein, P. M.: The seat belt syndrome. J. Trauma, 2:220-238, 1962.
Gibbens, M. E., Smith, W. V., and Studt, W. B.: The doctor and the automobile accident. J.A.M.A., 163:255-260, 1957.

Goddard, J. L.: Prevention of trauma: A joint responsibility. Amer. J. Surg., *95*:718-720, 1958.

Skudder, P. A., and Wade, P. A.: The organization of emergency medical facilities and service. J. Trauma, *4*:358-372, 1964.

Tobins, S. H.: An unusual injury due to the seat belt. J. Trauma, *4*:397-399, 1964.

Wade, P. A.: The responsibility of the medical profession to the victims of the automobile accident. Amer. J. Surg., *98*:526-529, 1959.

Watkins, G. L.: Blunt trauma to abdomen. Arch. Surg., *80*:187-191, 1960.

Wilson, D. H.: Incidence, aetiology, diagnosis and prognosis of closed abdominal injuries. A study of 265 cases. Brit. J. Surg., *50*:381-389, 1961.

2

RADIOGRAPHIC EXAMINATION

EVALUATION OF THE PATIENT

In the emergency room the physician makes an immediate and rapid medical evaluation of the patient by history and physical examination. He looks specifically for life-threatening injuries, quickly corrects interference with respiration, stops bleeding, supports the circulation and immobilizes obvious fractures. Blood is drawn for typing, cross-match and laboratory study. When the patient's general condition has stabilized, it is practical to proceed with the radiographic examination.

To plan his examination intelligently, the radiologist must know how the injury was incurred and what part of the abdomen sustained the blow. If this information cannot be obtained from the patient, the policeman or ambulance attendant, the detection of bruises, fractures and bleeding is helpful.

Bruises

External marks on the body show the site of the impact. For example, a bruise over the left upper abdomen indicates possible damage to the spleen (Figs. 2.1 and 2.2).

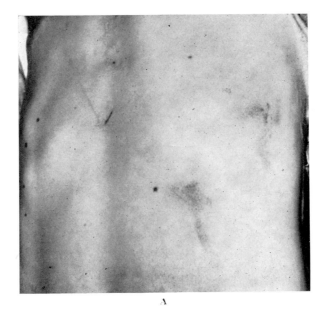

A

B

FIGURE 2.1. EXTERNAL SIGNS OF SITE OF IMPACT

A, Left upper quadrant bruises. C.D., a 13-year-old boy, fell from his bicycle. The site of impact is indicated by two large ecchymotic and abraded areas over the left anterior lower rib cage. Radiographically, there was blood in the peritoneal cavity and dilatation of the stomach. *B,* Specimen of spleen. The lower half of the spleen is almost completely transected.

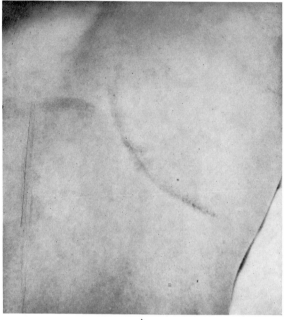

A

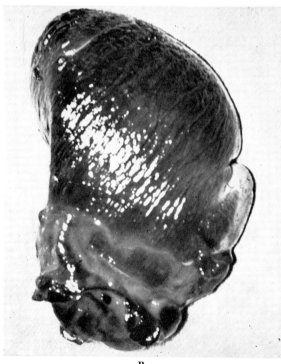

B

**FIGURE 2.2. EXTERNAL
SIGNS OF SITE OF
IMPACT.**

A, Horseshoe print. D.C.,
a 17-year-old boy, was
kicked in the left upper
abdomen by a horse. He
had generalized abdominal
pain associated with nau-
sea and vomiting. Radio-
graphic examination of the
abdomen and pneumoperi-
toneography showed peri-
splenic and intraperitoneal
hemorrhage. *B,* Specimen
of the spleen. A blood clot
had formed over this lacerated spleen and there was
free blood within the peritoneal cavity.

Fractures

Fractures of the skeleton supporting and surrounding the abdomen also suggest visceral injury. With lower rib fractures, the radiologist must suspect laceration of the liver or spleen (Fig. 2.3) ; with fractures of the transverse processes of the lumbar vertebrae, he must suspect injury to the kidney and ureters; and with fractures of the pelvis, he must suspect laceration of the bladder and urethra.

Bleeding

In addition, the radiologist must know whether the patient is bleeding from one of the natural orifices. Stomach contents are checked for blood by naso-gastric tube aspiration.[8] The stool and rectum are examined for blood. Urinalysis is done in every case and if the patient cannot void spontaneously, a catheterized specimen is obtained. If the patient is unconscious, the underclothing is examined for blood.

RADIOGRAPHIC TECHNIQUE

In handling the severely injured, movement is kept to a minimum. Radiographic equipment installed in the emergency area allows the patient to be examined in various projections without moving him to the x-ray department. A physician is in constant attendance when the severely injured patient is examined so that observation and support are continued while the radiographs are taken and processed.[3]

In the emergency radiographic area it has been found useful to have a ceiling-mounted tube combined with a wall-mounted Bucky stand (Fig. 2.4).

Guerneys with radiolucent backing can be rolled directly over a radiographic table or over a horizontal Bucky tray. Portable units can be used, but better films are made with a Bucky apparatus. A high grid ratio (i.e., 16:1) reduces scatter and gives optimum anatomic detail.

Since the tissues to be examined represent four degrees of density— bone, water (organ parenchyma and muscle), fat and air—the contrast between these structures is best shown at 60 to 70 kilovolts (Fig. 2.5).[5]

To keep the radiographic exposure time to a minimum, particularly if the patient is comatose or uncooperative, a high milliamperage (300 to 500) and high speed screens and film are needed. To reduce the patient's radiation exposure per film, an adjustable rectangular cone and 3 mm. of aluminum filtration are used. To produce optimum clarity and contrast the radiographs are developed according to the time and temperature recommendations of the film manufacturer.

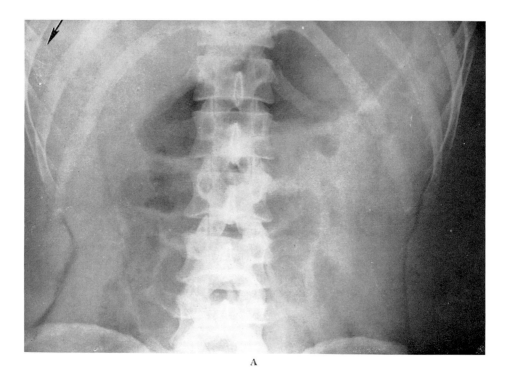

A

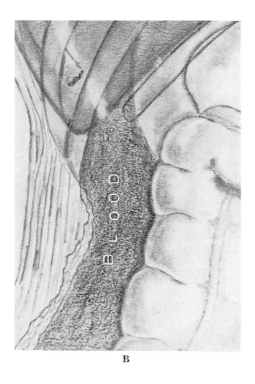

B

Figure 2.3. *See opposite page for legend.*

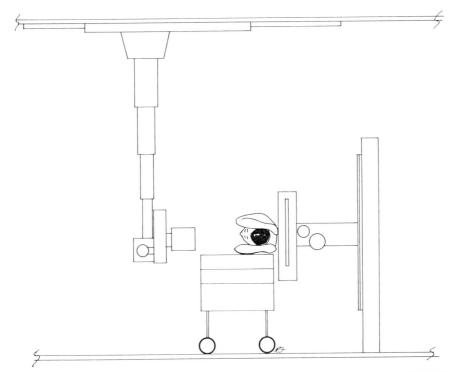

FIGURE 2.4. POSITION OF PATIENT FOR LATERAL DECUBITUS EXAMINATION OF ABDOMEN; RADIOGRAPHIC EQUIPMENT INSTALLED IN THE EMERGENCY AREA.

With an overhead tube and a wall-mounted Bucky apparatus, radiographs can be taken on the guerney in the supine and lateral decubitus projection with minimal movement of the patient. A 16:1 grid ratio is used. Exposures are made with 60 to 70 kilovolts, 300 milliamperes and the shortest possible time. A filter of 3 mm. Al is used and the beam is reduced to the exact size of the film by a rectangular diaphragm.

(Illustration on opposite page.)

FIGURE 2.3. RADIOGRAPHIC SIGNS OF THE SITE OF IMPACT: LIVER LACERATION.

A, Muscle contusion and fractured rib. A fracture through the right 7th rib anteriorly (arrow) is seen. Compare the right and left properitoneal fat lines. The right is irregular with swelling and thickening of the oblique abdominal muscles, and the lumbar spine is tilted to the right side. *B,* Diagram. The combination of the right lower rib fracture with contusion of the abdominal muscle shows that the major force of the blow was over the liver. (From McCort, J. J.: Rupture or laceration of the liver by nonpenetrating trauma. Radiology, *78:*49-57, 1962.)

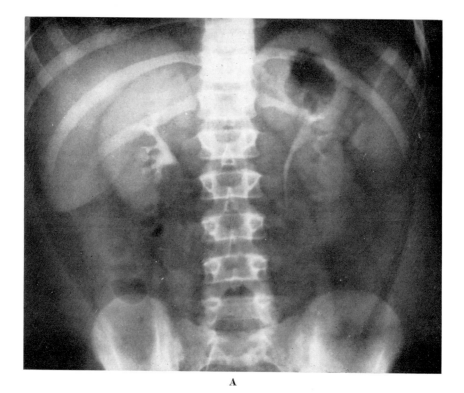

A

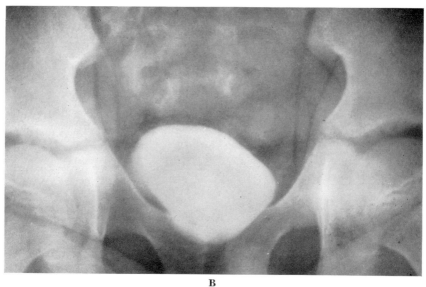

B

**FIGURE 2.5. NORMAL VISCERAL OUTLINES; CONTRAST OF ORGANS
WITH SURROUNDING FAT.**

A, Upper abdomen. In this young, obese, uninjured male, the lower margins
of the liver and spleen are shown by the contrast of the adjacent mesenteric fat.
Perinephric fat outlines the kidney. The lateral wall of the colon is visualized
against the extraperitoneal fat and the medial wall by the mesenteric fat. *B,*
Lower abdomen. The outer wall of the bladder is demarcated by perivesical fat.

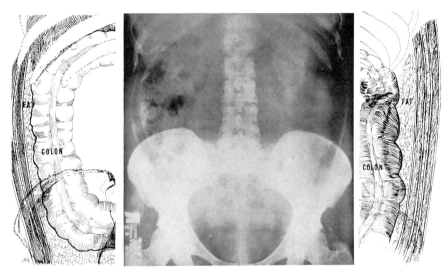

FIGURE 2.6. NORMAL RELATIONSHIP OF ASCENDING AND DESCENDING SEGMENTS OF COLON TO PERITONEAL FAT.

The segments of the colon are identified because they contain food residues and gas and show transverse haustral markings. Along the lateral margins, the colon indents the properitoneal fat. For adequate study in blunt abdominal trauma, both fat lines should be identified on the film.

The supine anteroposterior film of the abdomen gives most informa-tion. When indicated, additional films are taken with the patient in the lateral decubitus, oblique and prone positions. An upright view of the abdomen is desirable, but is often impossible to obtain with an injured patient.

In the study of the abdomen, the lower margin of the film includes the pelvic bones down to the ischia. Laterally, it includes both peritoneal fat lines in the flanks (Figs. 2.6 and 2.7). The reason for this is more fully discussed in Chapter 3. If, because of obesity, the entire abdomen is not covered on a single film, one should take two 14-by-17 films crosswise or increase the target-film distance to five or six feet. *A complete and satis-factory examination of the abdomen in blunt trauma requires that the lateral peritoneal fat lines be shown on the film.*

Films of the chest are taken routinely because the abdominal and thoracic viscera are contiguous and it is not uncommon to find injuries to both. Contusion of the lung, pneumo- and hemothorax or rupture of the diaphragm may be overlooked if the chest is not examined. The chest film also establishes a baseline position of the diaphragm for com-parison should injuries to the liver and spleen later manifest themselves by diaphragmatic elevation and limitation of motion.[1]

Radiographs of the supporting structures, the lower ribs, the lumbar

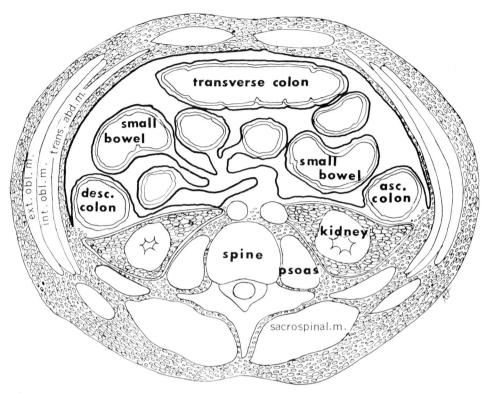

FIGURE 2.7. CROSS SECTION DIAGRAM: PERITONEAL REFLECTIONS.

The reflections of the peritoneal membrane limit the spread of blood after abdominal trauma. The site of the bleeding, whether intra- or retroperitoneal, depends on the location of the injured viscus. Note that the normal anatomical location of the ascending and descending segments of the colon is in the flanks and the lateral margins of the colon are adjacent to the properitoneal fat.

spine, the pelvis and hips are obtained when there are pain, deformity, limited motion and crepitation.

STUDY OF VISCERAL OUTLINES

Because the solid organs are surrounded totally (kidneys) or partially (bladder, liver, spleen) by a relatively radiolucent envelope of fat, they can be visualized on the plain film (Fig. 2.5). Satisfactory radiographic and film processing techniques are essential. Since visualization of the organ contour depends on the encircling layers of fat tissue, it is maximum in the obese patient. The lumen of the intestinal tract is delineated by gas or food residues. Study of the films with a spotlight of variable intensity aids identification.

Table 2.1. Distribution of Abdominal Injuries

	SOLHEIM[9]	MARTIN ET AL.[4]	WATKINS[10]	FITZGERALD[2]	WILSON[12]	MORTON ET AL.[*6]	KLEINERT[3]	WILLIAMS & ZOLLINGER[10]	SLÁTIS[†7]	MCCORT
Kidney	36.6%	36.1%	5.7%	3.1%	40%	29.9%	21.6%	27.8%[†]	23.0%	15.8%
Spleen	21.3	19.3	39.8	32.0	26.3	42.5	28.0	15.0	12.6	20.6
Liver	19.7	12.0	5.0	36.1	15.8		12.7	7.3	39.2	16.6
G.I. { Stomach		1.3		0.7					3.0	1.2
G.I. { Sm. bowel	8.2	9.5	9.9	6.2	9.5	15.0	6.9	24.6	3.0	12.6
G.I. { Colon	2.5	2.5		3.4						3.2
Diaphragm	4.1		0.7	5.5		4.6	2.9			4.5
Urinary bladder	3.3	15.5	7.8	2.7	3.1		15.7	21.2		6.9
Pancreas	2.2	2.8	2.8	0.7		2.3		4.9		4.9
Hemorrhage without visceral injury	2.2					2.3			4.4	4.0
Adrenal	1.4						3.4			
Gallbladder	1.0	0.9		0.3						
Mesentery			1.4	5.5			4.9		13.3	6.5
Abdominal wall			27.0	1.4		3.4				0.4
Uterus										0.8
Vascular				1.4			2.5		1.5	2.0
Urethra										
Miscellaneous				1.0			1.5			
Total injuries	366	316	141	291	95	87	201	273	135	247

* Plus 32 multiple severe injuries.
† Includes bladder.
‡ Autopsies only.

DISTRIBUTION OF ABDOMINAL INJURIES

In Table 2.1 are given the relative frequencies in which abdominal organs are injured according to large reported series. Considerable variation is apparent, depending on the method and criteria of selection. Intraperitoneally, the spleen is the most frequently injured organ; retroperitoneally, the kidney is most frequently injured. Blunt abdominal trauma is found in both sexes at any age. Young adult males are the most frequent victims because of greater occupational exposure and because they are more often involved in automobile accidents.[9, 13]

REFERENCES

1. Cimmino, C. V.: Ruptured spleen. Some refinements in its roentgenologic diagnosis. Radiology, 82:57-62, 1964.
2. Fitzgerald, J. B., Crawford, E. S., and DeBakey, M.: Surgical considerations of non-penetrating abdominal injuries. Amer. J. Surg., 100:22-29, 1960.
3. Kleinert, H. E., and Romero, J.: Blunt abdominal trauma. Review of cases admitted to a general hospital over a 10-year period. J. Trauma, 1:226-247, 1961.
4. Martin, J. D., Perdu, G. D., and Harrison, W. H.: Abdominal visceral injury due to non-penetrating trauma. A.M.A. Arch. Surg., 80:192-197, 1960.
5. Morgan, R. H.: Roentgen tube potential in diagnostic roentgenology. Amer. J. Roentgenol., 58:211-221, 1947.
6. Morton, J. H., Hinshaw, J. R., and Morton, J. J.: Blunt trauma to the abdomen. Ann. Surg., 145:699-711, 1957.
7. Slätis, P.: Injuries in fatal traffic accidents. An analysis of 349 medicolegal autopsies. Acta Chir. Scand., Suppl. 297, Stockholm, 1962.
8. Smith, G. K.: Diagnosis and management of blunt trauma to the abdomen. J. Occup. Med., 4:126-129, 1962.
9. Solheim, K.: Closed abdominal injuries. Acta Chir. Scand., 126:574-592, 1963.
10. Watkins, G. L.: Blunt trauma to the abdomen. Arch. Surg., 80:187-191, 1960.
11. Williams, R. D., and Zollinger, R. M.: Diagnostic and prognostic factors in abdominal trauma. Amer. J. Surg., 97:575-578, 1959.
12. Wilson, D. H.: Incidence, aetiology, diagnosis and prognosis of closed abdominal injuries. Brit. J. Surg., 50:381-389, 1961.
13. Woodruff, J. H., Ottoman, R. E., Simonton, J. H., and Averbrook, B. D.: Radiologic differential diagnosis of abdominal trauma. Radiology, 82:57-62, 1964.

3

RADIOGRAPHIC SIGNS
OF ABDOMINAL INJURY

DISRUPTION OF SUPPORTING STRUCTURES

Radiographic signs of abdominal injury consist of fractures of the lower ribs, lumbosacral spine and pelvis, and contusions of the extraperitoneal fat and abdominal muscles.

Fracture of Lower Ribs, Lumbosacral Spine and Pelvis

Since the techniques of examination and the radiographic changes are well known, they will not be discussed here. *Certain visceral injuries are more likely in the presence of fracture (e.g., bladder injury is found in one of ten patients with low pelvic fracture).* The radiologist must be alert to these possibilities and should initiate the studies necessary to evaluate concomitant visceral injury.

Contusion of Extraperitoneal Fat

Hemorrhage into the extraperitoneal fat and the fat between the muscle planes results in a loss of normal radiolucency. The density of the fat approaches that of the adjacent muscle (Fig. 3.1). Consequently, the extraperitoneal fat lines at the site of injury are distorted, fragmented or obliterated.

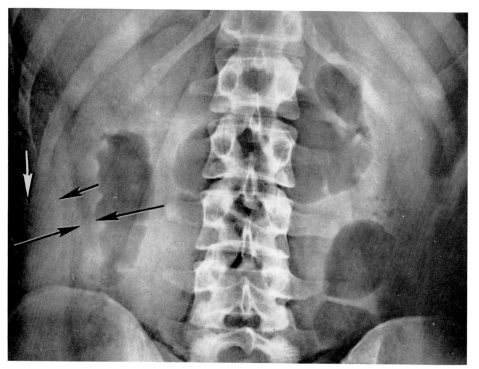

FIGURE 3.1. CONTUSION OF RIGHT OBLIQUE ABDOMINAL MUSCLES AND EXTRAPERITONEAL FAT; HEMOPERITONEUM; LIVER LACERATION.

R.A. had fractures of the right 3rd to 7th ribs with a small amount of blood in the pleural space. On the abdominal film the right oblique and transverse abdominal muscles are thickened and shortened (short arrows) and the adjacent properitoneal fat is irregular (long arrows). Contusion of the extraperitoneal fat and abdominal muscles shows the site of impact. Blood is present in the peritoneal cavity from a laceration of the right lobe of the liver.

Abdominal Muscle Injury

The muscles enclosing the abdomen are invariably injured in blunt trauma and the spectrum of injury ranges from mild contusion to complete transection. Usually these muscular injuries are overshadowed by the concomitant visceral damage.

On clinical examination muscle contusion is manifest by tenderness, spasm and echymoses.

Injury in the larger muscles, such as the psoas, the internal oblique, external oblique and obturator internus may be visible radiographically. The contused muscle is thickened, irregular and shortened because of intra muscular hemorrhage and reflex spasm (Fig. 3.1). With abdominal muscle injury, there may be a scoliosis of the lumbar spine concave toward the injured side. The presence of muscle injury points to the site of impact in the unconscious patient. Diaphragmatic laceration is described separately (Chapter 11).

ALTERATION OF VISCERAL OUTLINE

Injury alters the visceral outline in three ways: loss of outline, displacement and enlargement. These changes are usually the result of hemorrhage and are discussed more fully under that heading.

Loss of Outline

Hemorrhage or exudate infiltrates the radiolucent fat around an organ and obscures its outline. This finding is most useful when a paired organ, such as a kidney, is injured and comparison with the uninjured side is made (Fig. 3.2).

Anatomic Displacement of Abdominal Organs

Displacement of the abdominal organs is strikingly seen with diaphragmatic rupture. At times the spleen, stomach, small bowel and portions of the colon or liver may extrude into the left thorax. When an organ is enlarged by intraparenchymal or subcapsular hemorrhage, it will displace adjacent viscera. This is commonly seen in splenic injury.

Gross Enlargement

Solid organs are enlarged by intraparenchymal and subcapsular hemorrhages. This is found in liver, spleen and kidney injury. Subcapsular hematoma gives the solid viscus a nodular outline; intraparenchymal hemorrhage and edema produce diffuse enlargement.

HEMORRHAGE

Blunt injury to the abdomen causes hemorrhage of varying degree. The amount of bleeding depends on the size and number of the torn vessels, as well as on the efficiency of the hemostatic mechanisms. With minor injury, the bleeding is slight; within a short time the blood is absorbed and the patient has no further symptoms.

When bleeding continues, clinical signs of blood loss appear. Radiographic changes depend on the amount of blood lost and its location. The bleeding may be (1) subcapsular or subserosal, (2) localized to the area

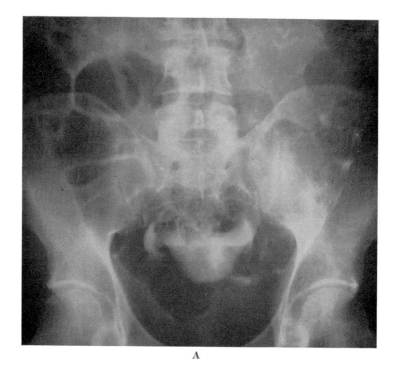

A

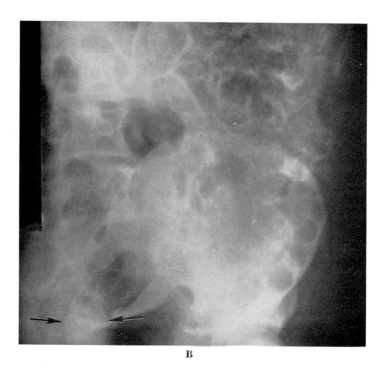

B

Figure 3.2. *Legend on opposite page*

occupied by the organ, (3) free in the peritoneal cavity, or (4) retroperitoneal. The location of the bleeding shows whether the injured organ is intra- or retroperitoneal.

In recent years the four quadrant abdominal tap has been used to detect intraperitoneal bleeding. In an experiment with 80 dogs subjected to abdominal trauma, Baxter and Williams[1] found that needle aspiration was positive in 90 per cent of the animals. Williams and Zollinger[8] demonstrated the four quadrant tap to be 79 per cent accurate. There were two false positive and three false negative examinations.

In the experience of the author, an adequate radiographic examination is more reliable in the detection of abdominal bleeding than the physical examination or the exploratory needle puncture. It is usually possible to distinguish between intra- and extraperitoneal bleeding radiographically, but this is difficult or impossible by needle tap (Fig. 9.8).

The diagnostic abdominal tap complements the radiographic examination. It is indicated when the radiographic examination is equivocal or is not consistent with clinical and laboratory evidence of blood loss.

Subcapsular or Subserosal Hemorrhage

In the liver and spleen, subcapsular hemorrhage causes a localized bulge in the organ contour with a displacement of adjacent viscera.[6] Usually, the outline of the organ remains intact. If the plain film diagnosis is not clear, the radiologist can employ special procedures (Chapter 4). When bleeding is limited, a small subcapsular hematoma is absorbed. With continuous bleeding, the capsule over the hematoma will become thin and eventually will rupture; a large amount of blood then pours into the peritoneal cavity. This is one theory of the mechanism for delayed bleeding and shock. In a few cases the hematoma liquefies and a pseudocyst develops.

Subserosal and intramural hemorrhages alter the contour of the hollow muscular organs such as the bowel, by encroaching on the lumen. Usually this is not detectable on the plain film and opacification studies are needed.

(Illustration on opposite page.)

FIGURE 3.2. FILLING OF PELVIC RECESSES; DIATRIZOATE INJECTED INTO PERITONEUM.

A, Anteroposterior. J.A., a young man, had been stabbed in the abdomen. To determine whether the peritoneum had been opened, 30 milliliters of 50 percent diatrizoate sodium was injected along the knife track. The opaque medium entered the peritoneum. *B,* Oblique. The contrast medium lies mainly in the space between the rectum and bladder, the pouch of Douglas (arrows).

Localized Hemorrhage

Bleeding can be localized to the fossa containing the kidney or spleen. When the fossa is completely filled with blood, the normal sharp outline of the organ is replaced by a poorly circumscribed homogeneous density and adjacent viscera are pushed aside.

Intraperitoneal Hemorrhage

With continued hemorrhage due to tearing of large vessels, the peritoneal cavity fills with blood. When the patient is supine, blood in the peritoneal cavity gravitates into the flanks and pelvis.[3] Usually the pelvic recesses fill first and the early signs of hemorrhage are found in the pelvis (Figs. 3.2 and 3.3).

Accumulation of Blood in the Pelvis

Blood in the pelvis fills the pouch of Douglas and the peritoneal recesses on each side of the bladder and rectum (Fig. 3.4). This blood appears as a density above and lateral to the bladder. Blood in the pelvis has the same density as the urine-filled bladder. It is seen separate from the bladder because of the intervening layer of extraperitoneal, perivesical fat (Fig. 3.6). Extending superiorly above the bladder, it resembles the projecting ears of a dog, the "dog's ears" sign (Figs. 3.5 and 3.6).

In addition to the site of the trauma, the position of the patient following the injury (whether he is lying on the right or left side) influences the location of the free blood (Fig. 3.7). Thus, at times, more blood will be found in one flank or one side of the pelvis.

DIFFERENTIAL DIAGNOSIS OF BLOOD IN THE PELVIS. Two conditions simulate blood in the pelvis: fluid filled small bowel loops and pelvic tumor.

Fluid-filled Loops of Small Bowel in the Pelvis. Because they appear as a density above the bladder, fluid-filled loops of small bowel resemble free intraperitoneal blood in the pelvis (Fig. 3.8). When the margins of the fluid-filled loops are visible, the characteristic sausage shape and distribution of small bowel loops differentiate them from free blood. Furthermore, they do not have the homogeneous density seen with blood alone. In questionable cases, oral contrast media can be used to outline the small bowel.

Pelvic Tumor. Pelvic tumors are found predominantly in the female patient and are of uterine or ovarian origin. At times, an early gravid or postpartum uterus presents a differential problem. Radiographically, pelvic tumors will indent the roof of the bladder, whereas blood in the

(*Text continued on page 27*)

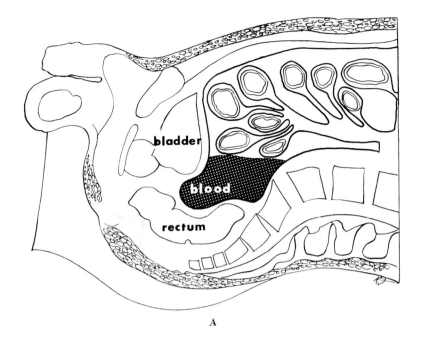

A

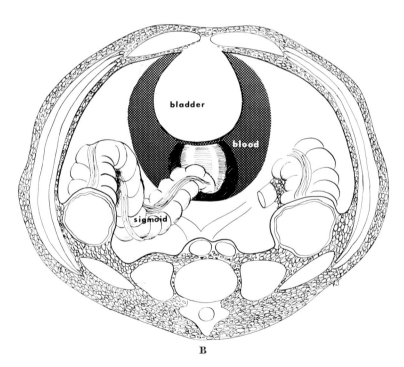

B

FIGURE 3.3. DIAGRAM: BLOOD IN THE PELVIS.

A, Sagittal section. Blood gravitates to the pelvis, the lowest part of the peritoneal cavity when the patient is supine. *B*, Cross section. Blood in the pelvis is
equally distributed on both sides of the bladder and rectum unless the patient
has been lying on one side. When the lateral recesses of the bladder and rectum
are filled by blood, the small bowel is displaced out of the pelvis.

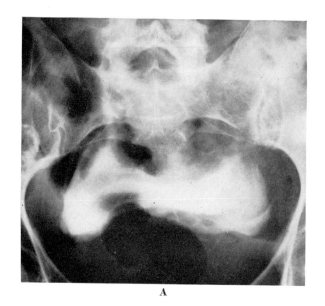

A

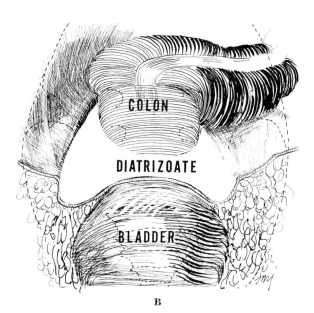

B

**FIGURE 3.4.   FLUID IN PELVIS; ASCITIC FLUID TAGGED WITH DIATRIZOATE;
"DOG'S EARS SIGN."**

A, Anteroposterior. M.K. had nutritional cirrhosis with ascites. Fifty milliliters of ascitic fluid were removed and replaced with an equivalent amount of diatrizoate.   *B,* Diagram. Diatrizoate in the pelvic recesses on either side of the bladder and rectum.

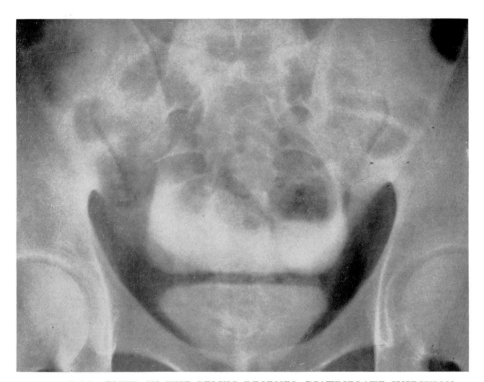

FIGURE 3.5. FLUID IN THE PELVIC RECESSES; DIATRIZOATE INJECTION.

R. C. was admitted with a self-inflicted knife wound. Sixty milliliters of 50 per cent diatrizoate were injected. That the wound communicated with the peritoneal cavity is shown by the accumulation of diatrizoate in the pelvic recesses. A simultaneous intravenous urogram opacified the bladder.

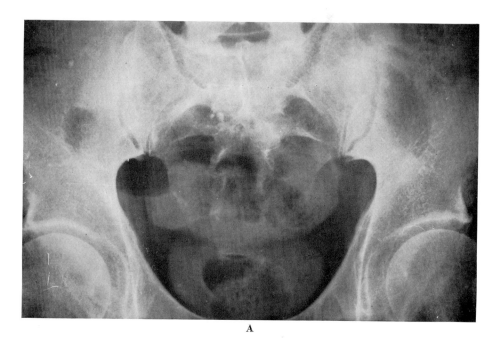

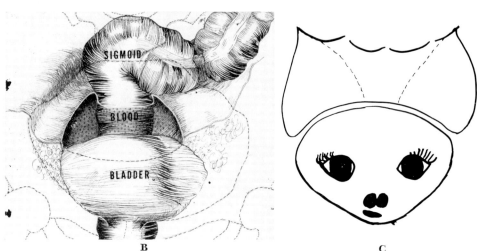

FIGURE 3.6. BLOOD IN THE PELVIS; THE "DOG'S EARS SIGN."

A, Anteroposterior. H.C. was thrown from his car, and his spleen was broken into three fragments. In the supine position, free blood in the peritoneum gravitates to the dependent pelvic recesses on both sides of the rectum and bladder. *B,* Diagram. Blood in pelvic recesses.   *C,* Diagram. "Dog's ears."

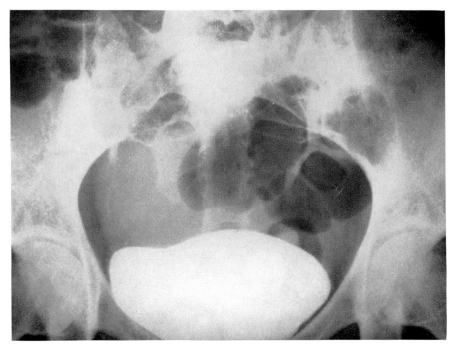

**FIGURE 3.7. LACERATION OF THE SPLEEN; BLOOD IN
OPPOSITE SIDE OF THE PELVIS.**

J. H. had a fracture of the left 7th rib posteriorly and a splenic mass. Blood
in the right side of the pelvis has displaced the colon and small bowel to the
left. Also, there is a slight indentation of the roof of the bladder by the uterus.
The unilateral localization of the blood occurred because the patient found
it less painful to lie on the right side following injury.

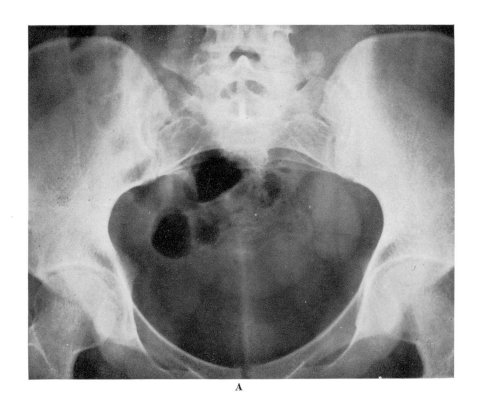

A

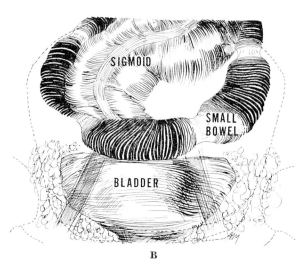

B

FIGURE 3.8. SMALL BOWEL LOOPS SIMULATING FLUID IN PELVIS.

A, In this uninjured patient, normal small bowel loops simulate free fluid. *B,* These loops have a sausage-like pattern. They are not homogeneous and do not fill the pelvic recesses as does fluid.

pelvis does not do so (Fig. 3.9). If the bladder is not seen, it is made visible by water soluble iodide or air. The superior margin of a pelvic tumor is smooth, sharply outlined and convex upward, whereas blood in the pelvis is not sharply outlined and extends laterally upward along the flanks. The differentiation can be definitively made by pneumoperitoneography (Chapter 4).

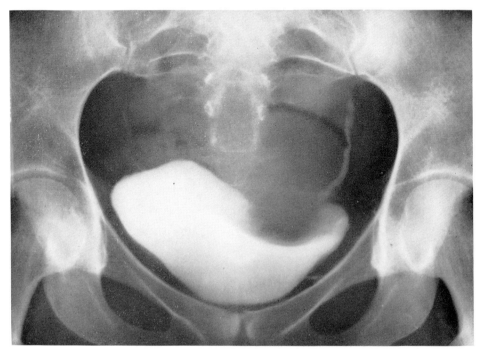

FIGURE 3.9. POSTPARTUM UTERUS SIMULATING FLUID IN THE PELVIS.

This 35-year-old multiparous woman was three months postpartum. There had been no trauma and the intravenous urogram was done because of a kidney infection. The upper margin of the uterus is outlined by gas-filled small bowel; it is smooth and convex cranially. Pelvic tumor indents the bladder and intraperitoneal blood does not. When blood in the pelvis is suspected, the bladder is emptied and cystography is done.

Accumulation of Blood in the Flanks

The peritoneal membrane is too thin to be identified on the radiograph. However, the layer of fat (the extraperitoneal or properitoneal fat) which lies between the peritoneum and transverse abdominal muscles can be seen on the plain film and defines the outer surface of the peritoneum. Ordinarily, the ascending and descending portions of the colon lie adjacent to the inner surface of the peritoneal membrane. The colon is shown radiographically when it contains gas and feces. (Gas is introduced when

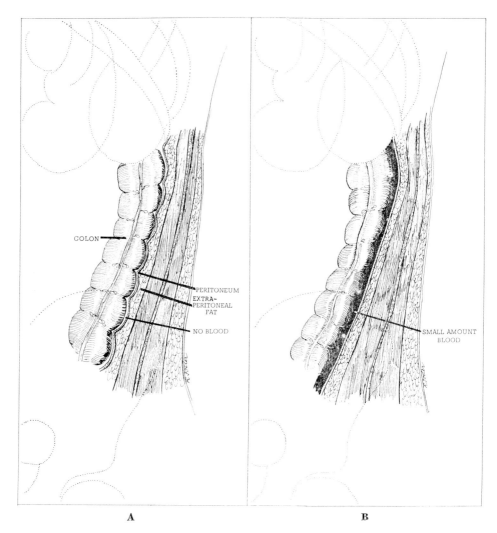

A   B

FIGURE 3.10. DIAGRAM: SIGNS OF FLUID IN FLANK.

A, The normal relationship of the wall of the colon, the peritoneum and the
extraperitoneal fat. *B,* With a small amount of blood, the conformation of the
fat to the haustra is lost. *C,* Increasing amounts of blood form a band of density between the gas-filled colon and the extraperitoneal fat. The blood also
projects between the haustra.
(After Laurell[5] and Frimann-Dahl.[3])

the colon is not visible [Chapter 4].) Hence, the only radiographic structure
lying between the radiolucent colonic gas and the outer surface of the
peritoneum is the lateral wall of the colon, a thin layer of fluid and the
peritoneum. In the absence of bleeding, the properitoneal fat conforms
to the haustra of the colon so that the interface between colon and fat
is nodular in outline (Fig. 3.10).

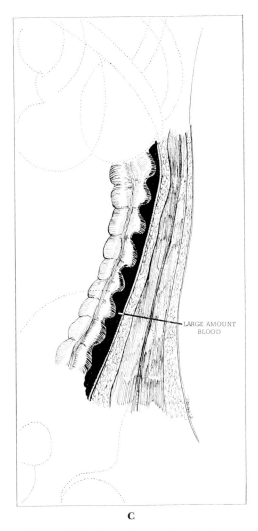

LARGE AMOUNT
BLOOD

C

Figure 3.10. *Legend on opposite page.*

In 1935, H. Laurell[5] pointed out that when the fluid between the colon and properitoneal fat increases, the conformation of the fat layer to the colon disappears and the interface between colon and fat becomes smooth. This is an early sign and is present with a small amount of blood (Fig. 3.10).

As the amount of blood in the paracolic gutter increases, the colon is displaced more medially (Fig. 3.10). On the radiograph, a band of increased density representing free blood is interposed between the gas-filled colon and properitoneal fat (Figs. 3.11 and 3.12). The blood extends into the spaces formed by the haustra (Figs. 3.13, 3.14, 3.15 and 3.16). Laurell[5] described comblike projections when the fluid extends between coiled loops of small bowel. An excellent description of the radiographic changes found with fluid in the flanks or pelvis is given by Frimann-Dahl.[3]

(Text continued on page 34)

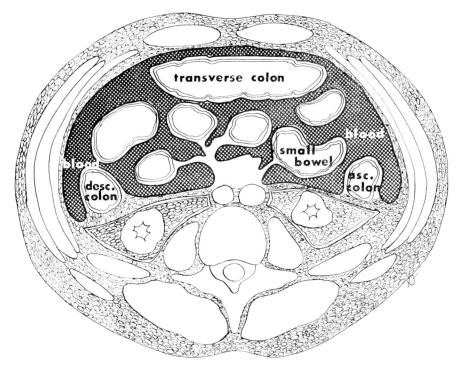

**FIGURE 3.11.   DIAGRAM: MASSIVE INTRAPERITONEAL HEMORRHAGE;
CROSS-SECTION.**

In the flanks, the blood is interposed between the properitoneal fat and the
ascending and descending segments of the colon. These segments are displaced
medially by the blood. Small bowel loops float toward the midline. The kidneys
are not obscured because the perirenal fat is intact.

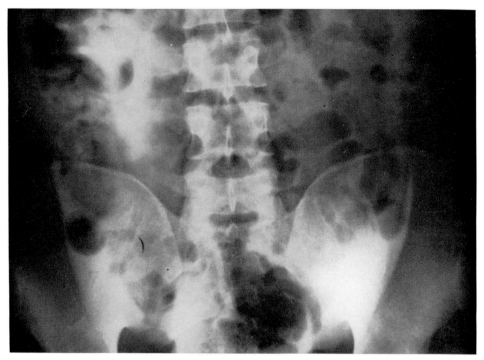

**FIGURE 3.12. FLUID IN THE FLANKS BETWEEN THE COLON
AND THE PROPERITONEAL FAT.**

R.C. was admitted with a self-inflicted knife wound (Fig. 3.5). Sixty milliliters of 50 percent diatrizoate sodium were injected into the wound to see whether it communicated with the peritoneum. The injected diatrizoate is seen in the peritoneal cavity between the colon and properitoneal fat.

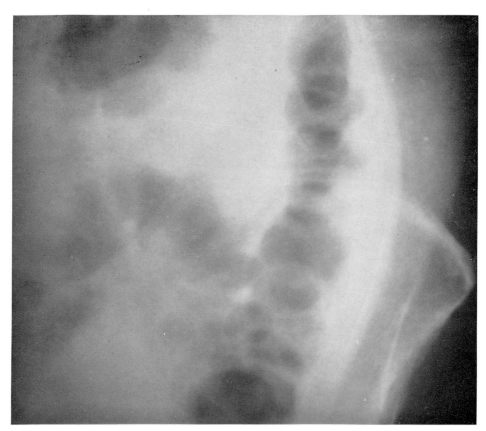

FIGURE 3.13. FLUID IN FLANK; ASCITIC FLUID OPACIFIED BY DIATRIZOATE.

N.H. a 50-year-old woman, had nutritional cirrhosis and ascites. Five hundred milliliters of ascitic fluid were removed and 120 milliliters of 50 percent diatrizoate sodium injected. Opacified ascitic fluid fills the space between the colon and fat line.

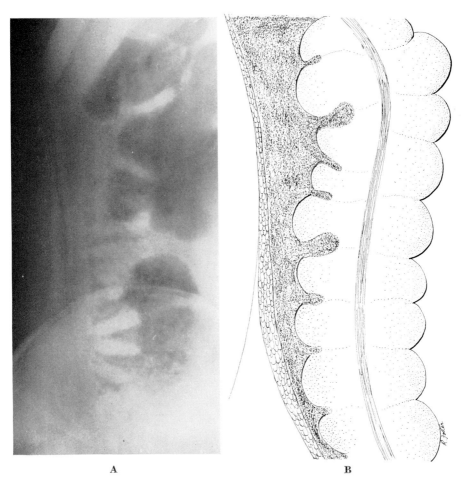

A   B

**FIGURE 3.14. BLOOD IN THE RIGHT FLANK BETWEEN
COLON AND EXTRAPERITONEAL FAT.**

A, Plain film. L.C., a 15-year-old girl, had been in an automobile accident.
There is blood between the colon and the extraperitoneal fat. *B,* Diagram. A
ruptured spleen and about 500 milliliters of free blood were found at operation.
(Courtesy of Justin R. Colburn, M.D., San Leandro, California.)

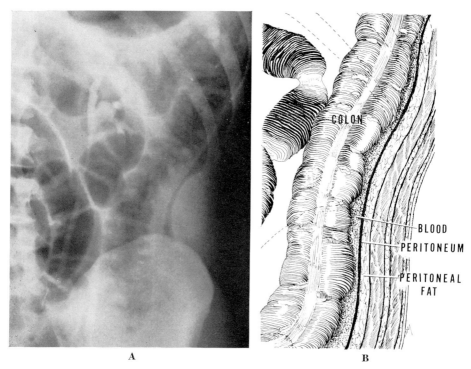

A   B

FIGURE 3.15. BLOOD IN THE LEFT FLANK BETWEEN THE COLON AND EXTRAPERITONEAL FAT.

A, Anteroposterior film. J.M. was in shock and had a falling hematocrit after having been struck by a bus. A flattening of the inner margin of the extraperitoneal fat line is present and there is a density between the colon and the fat line. *B,* Diagram. At operation, there was considerable blood in the peritoneal cavity from a rupture of the spleen and a tear of the sigmoid mesentery.

As little as several hundred milliliters of blood may be detected when good roentgenographic technique allows visualization of the properitoneal fat lines.

DIFFERENTIAL DIAGNOSIS. Three conditions can simulate fluid in the flanks: (1) interposition of a loop of small bowel, (2) a low margin of the right lobe of the liver and (3) fluid within the ascending colon. The first is commonly seen on the left side, the latter two only on the right.

Interposition of a Loop of Small Bowel. A fluid-filled loop of small bowel, interposed between the colon and properitoneal fat line, appears as a density simulating free blood (Fig. 3.17), but there is no fluid in the opposite flank or pelvis. If the differentiation is not possible by this means, the radiologist can give the patient contrast media orally to outline the small bowel. Turning the patient may dislodge the interposed loop.

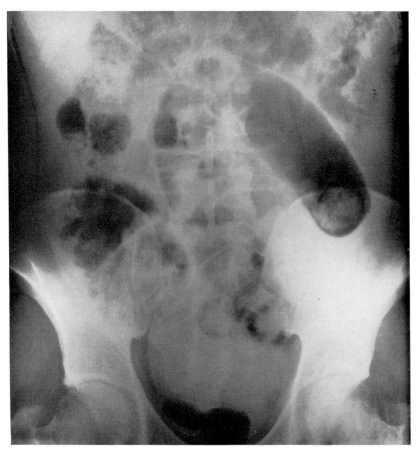

**FIGURE 3.16. MASSIVE HEMOPERITONEUM; BLOOD FILLING
FLANKS AND PELVIS.**

L.A., a 22-year-old man, had fractures of the right 5th and 9th ribs. After an
air enema, medial displacement of both the ascending and descending colon segments is shown. Blood lies between the colon and fat line bilaterally and fills
the pelvic recesses. At celiotomy, 2000 milliliters of fresh blood filled the peritoneal cavity from a liver laceration.

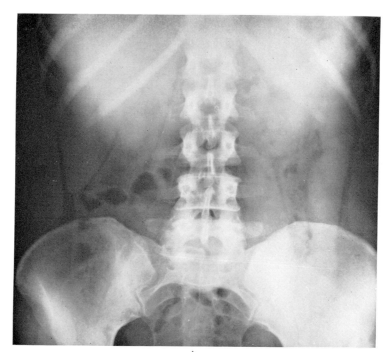

A

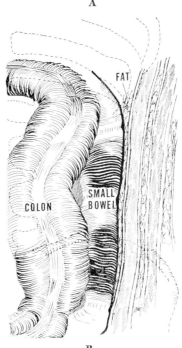

B

FIGURE 3.17. INTERPOSITION OF SMALL BOWEL LOOP SIMULATING BLOOD IN LEFT ABDOMEN.

A, Plain film. J.K. This patient had no injury. Free intraperitoneal fluid is simulated by a loop of small bowel in the left flank. However, there is an absence of fluid on the opposite side and in the pelvis. *B,* Diagram. Rotation of the patient tends to displace the loop of small bowel. Diatrizoate administered orally will outline the small bowel if interposition is suspected.

36

Low Liver Edge.   Occasionally, a low position of the right lobe of the liver causes medial displacement of the ascending colon and simulates fluid in the right gutter (Fig. 3.18).   The continuity of this density with the undersurface of the liver distinguishes it from intraperitoneal bleeding.

Fluid within the Cecum and Ascending Colon.   At times, and particularly in children, the contents of the cecum and ascending colon are liquid.   With both gas and fluid in the ascending colon, the bowel appears to be separated from the extraperitoneal fat and blood in the flank is suggested (Fig. 3.19).   When the patient is placed in the erect or lateral decubitus position, the true location of the fluid is apparent.   Intraperitoneal fluid is ruled out because this is seen only on the right side and there is no evidence of fluid in the left flank or pelvis.   The nodular conformation of the fat to the colon remains.

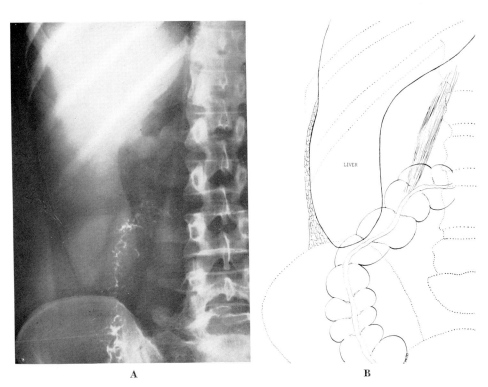

A   B

FIGURE 3.18.   RIGHT LOBE OF THE LIVER SIMULATING BLOOD IN THE RIGHT ABDOMEN.

A, Anteroposterior. J.C. This is the postevacuation film of a barium enema in an uninjured patient. A low extension of the right lobe of the liver is present with medial displacement of the ascending colon and hepatic flexure. *B,* Diagram. Because it forms a continuous shadow with the liver, this should not be mistaken for fluid in the right flank.

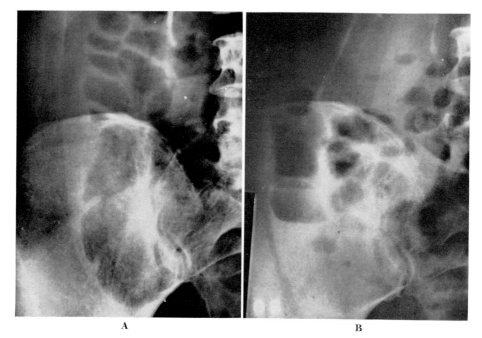

A   B

**FIGURE 3.19. FLUID IN THE ASCENDING COLON SIMULATING BLOOD IN THE
RIGHT ABDOMEN.**

A, Supine. R.O.N., a 36-year-old woman, had no trauma to the abdomen. On
this intravenous urogram there is a suggestion of fluid between the ascending
colon and properitoneal fat. *B,* Erect. The fluid is actually within the lumen of
the ascending colon. Note fluid levels. Liquid stool in the right colon can
follow cathartic administration.

Other Signs of Intraperitoneal Bleeding

In order of importance, other signs of free intraperitoneal bleeding
are: (1) flotation of gas-filled small bowel loop, (2) increased space between
small bowel loops and (3) image unsharpness.

Flotation of Small Bowel. Gas-filled loops of small bowel float to
the center of the abdomen in the supine film (Fig. 3.20).

Increased Space Between Loops. Small bowel loops are separated
by free blood. This simulates thickening of the bowel wall except that
the valvulae conniventes are not widened.

Image Unsharpness. Large amounts of intraperitoneal fluid produce
greater scattering of the incident x-ray beam, causing unsharpness of the
visceral outline and bone detail, the "ground-glass" appearance. This
change is produced by other factors which cause image unsharpness such
as motion of the patient, underexposure of the film or improper dark-
room procedures. Since a clinically obvious amount of fluid must be
present to produce significant scatter and loss of sharpness, this sign is of
little value.

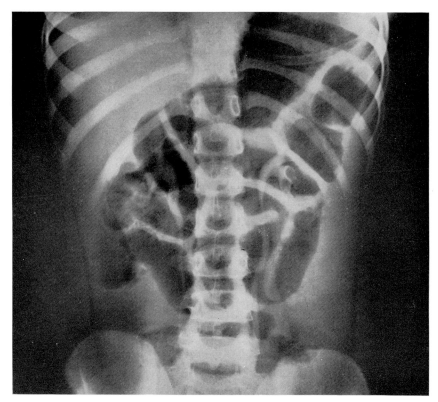

FIGURE 3.20. FLOTATION OF GAS-FILLED LOOPS OF SMALL BOWEL BY INTRAPERITONEAL HEMORRHAGE.

V.C. had fractures of both pubic bones. There is fluid in the flanks interposed between the colon and fat lines. On both sides the fat lines are smooth. Gas-filled loops of small bowel float on top of intraperitoneal blood and cluster in the middle of the abdomen. At celiotomy, the jejunum was found to be transected and bleeding freely.

Blood in the peritoneal cavity ordinarily will not obscure the outlines of the retroperitoneal structures such as the kidneys and psoas muscles (Fig. 8.2). If these structures are not seen on a well exposed film, then retroperitoneal injury is likely.

Retroperitoneal Bleeding

When retroperitoneal bleeding occurs, the injured viscera lose their normal outline and adjacent organs are displaced (Fig. 3.21). Perirenal hematoma obscures the outline of the kidney and ipsilateral psoas muscle. It displaces the overlying colon inferiorly and medially. Hemorrhage around the pancreas displaces the stomach and duodenum anteriorly. Hemorrhage filling the retroperitoneal structures of the pelvis deforms the bladder and rectum (Chapter 15).

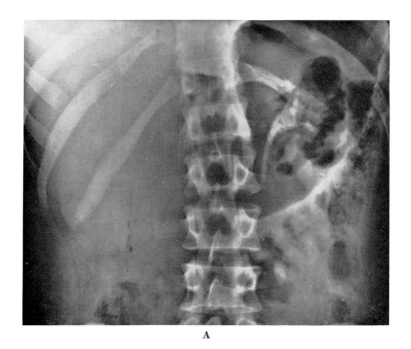

A

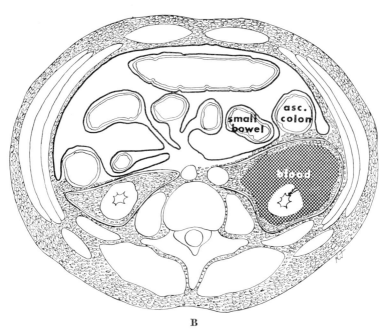

B

Figure 3.21. *Legend on opposite page.*

RUPTURE OF GAS-CONTAINING VISCERA

When gastrointestinal viscera rupture, gas and food residues escape into the peritoneal or retroperitoneal spaces. Stomach or colon perforation frequently gives rise to free air. Small bowel perforation only occasionally causes free air.[4]

Lateral Decubitus and Upright Projections

A decubitus or upright abdominal film with a horizontal beam is taken when possible. Free air accumulates beneath the diaphragm on the upright, and over the liver on the left lateral decubitus projection. If the patient can be examined only in the supine position, a cross-table lateral film with the x-ray beam horizontal will show air beneath the anterior abdominal wall. This projection is less satisfactory than the upright and decubitus positions.

Free air beneath the diaphragm appears as a radiolucent sickle-shaped shadow (Fig. 3.22). With the patient in the left lateral decubitus position, the air is found at the highest point between the liver and the right lateral abdominal wall (Fig. 3.23). To allow sufficient time for air to rise over the liver, the patient remains in the decubitus position for 10 to 15 minutes before the films are taken.

(Illustration on opposite page.)

FIGURE 3.21. RETROPERITONEAL BLEEDING OF RIGHT KIDNEY;
LOSS OF VISCERAL OUTLINE; DISPLACEMENT OF COLON.

A, Intravenous urogram. E.L. had rigidity of the entire right abdomen and grossly bloody urine. The right kidney shows no function and is obscured by a perirenal mass. The spine is tilted to the right. A badly lacerated right kidney was found and removed. *B,* Diagram. Retroperitoneal hemorrhage pushes the overlying small and large bowel loops against the curved anterior abdominal wall. On the anteroposterior radiograph, the displaced bowel lies inferiorly and medially to its normal anatomic position. An apparent density is seen between the displaced colon and the lateral properitoneal fat line and must not be confused with intraperitoneal blood.

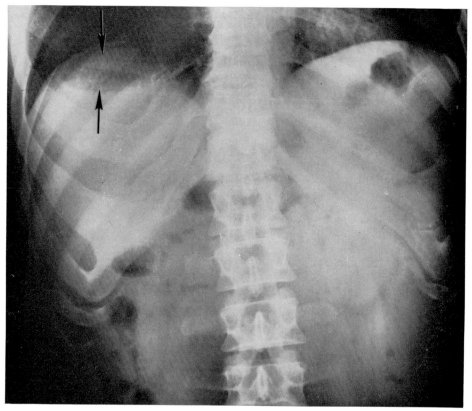

**FIGURE 3.22.   FREE AIR BENEATH THE RIGHT LEAF OF THE DIAPHRAGM;
PERFORATION OF THE JEJUNUM.**

R.J. had a boardlike rigidity of the abdomen, with diffuse tenderness and absence of peristalsis. On the erect film, free air (arrows) is present beneath the right leaf of the diaphragm. This had leaked from a one-inch laceration of the jejunum.

DIFFERENTIAL DIAGNOSIS OF FREE AIR. Two conditions mimic free air in the peritoneal cavity. One is the interposition of a gas-filled loop of bowel between the diaphragm and the liver. The other is the presence of extraperitoneal fat beneath the diaphragm or an irregularity of the diaphragm.

Interposition of Gas-filled Bowel. Interposed small bowel is identified by valvulae conniventes and the large bowel by haustra. With free air, a change in the patient's position (from erect to decubitus) causes displacement of gas on the radiograph (Fig. 3.24). This does not occur with interposition.

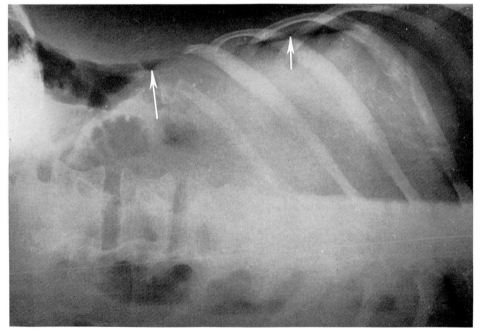

FIGURE 3.23. FREE AIR OVER THE LIVER; LEFT LATERAL DECUBITUS FILM; PERFORATION OF JEJUNUM.

R.W. had abdominal pain of 12 hours' duration after an automobile accident. With the patient's left side down, the radiograph is taken with the x-ray beam horizontal. Free air is seen over the right lobe (right arrow) and at the inferior tip of the liver (left arrow).

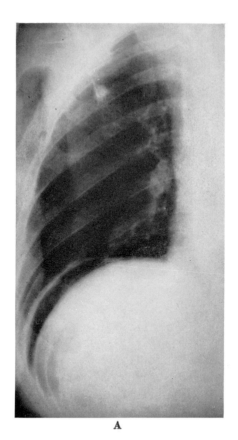

A

B

FIGURE 3.24. INTERPOSITION OF COLON BETWEEN DIAPHRAGM AND LIVER SIMULATING PNEUMOPERITONEUM.

A, Supine film. This elderly woman had no abdominal trauma. On the chest film, air is seen beneath the right leaf of the diaphragm. Perforation was suspected. *B,* Lateral decubitus film. The air is contained within the hepatic flexure of the colon, which is identified by haustral markings.

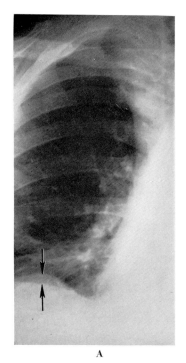
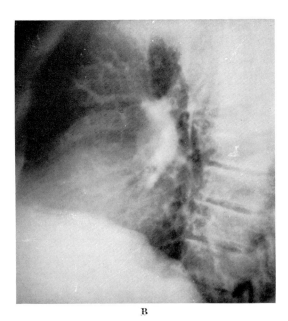

A   B

FIGURE 3.25. PSEUDOPNEUMOPERITONEUM; UNEVENNESS OF THE RIGHT LEAF OF THE DIAPHRAGM.

A, Anteroposterior chest. F.C., a 60-year-old man, had no abdominal complaint. The chest film shows a small semilunar radiolucency beneath the right leaf of the diaphragm (arrows). *B*, Right lateral chest. There is an unevenness of the right leaf of the diaphragm, and the superimposition of the ridges of the diaphragm simulates pneumoperitoneum.

Extraperitoneal Fat below Diaphragm or Irregular Diaphragm. Free air can be simulated by the presence of a fat pad (extraperitoneal fat) beneath the diaphragm or by an intrinsic irregularity of the diaphragm. Mokrohisky[7] has termed this appearance pseudopneumoperitoneum. In all 11 patients described by him, the left leaf of the diaphragm was involved. In making the differential diagnosis, it should be noted that the fat pad does not change when the position of the patient is altered (erect to lateral decubitus). A lateral film of the chest will demonstrate an irregularity of the diaphragm if this is the cause of the confusing shadow (Fig. 3.25).

Supine Projection

If films cannot be taken with a horizontal beam, the radiologist can find evidence of free air in the supine films (Fig. 3.25). Three helpful

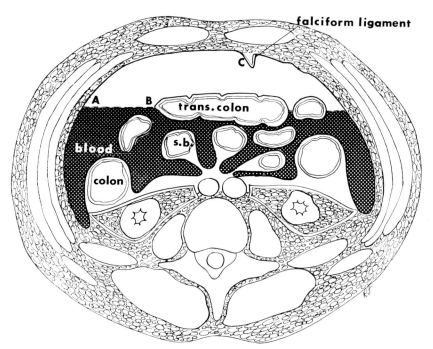

FIGURE 3.26.   DIAGRAM: CROSS-SECTION OF ABDOMEN; AIR AND BLOOD IN THE PERITONEAL SPACE; PATIENT SUPINE.

Air comes from perforation of the intestinal tract and fluid from the intestinal tract or torn vessels. With the patient supine, three characteristic signs are: (1) the dome or football sign, (2) air against the outside wall of the bowel, (3) air on both sides of the falciform ligament.

signs are: (1) the "dome" or "football" sign (Fig. 3.26*A*), (2) visualization of air against the outer walls of large or small bowel (Fig. 3.26*B*), and (3) delineation of the falciform ligament (Fig. 3.26*C*).

The Dome or Football Sign. The dome sign is seen when a large amount of both fluid and air is present in the peritoneal space. With the patient supine, the gas forms a dome or large bubble over the fluid and the circular margin of the gas-fluid interface is seen (Figs. 3.27 and 3.28).

Visualization of Air Against Outer Wall of Large or Small Bowel. Visualization of air against the outer wall of large or small bowel loops (Fig. 3.29) is possible when the loops are gas-filled. This can be simulated by two distended, gas-filled loops against each other. Hence this sign is most reliable when the outer wall of the bowel is seen adjacent to or over the liver (Fig. 3.30).

Delineation of the Falciform Ligament. The falciform ligament is formed by a double layer of peritoneum and derives from the primitive vascular structures of the embryo. Anatomically, it extends from the anterior-superior surface of the liver to the anterior abdominal wall.[2] The

(*Text continued on page 52*)

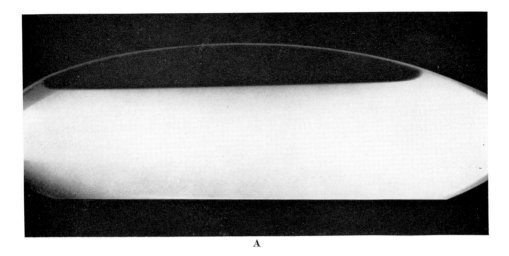

A

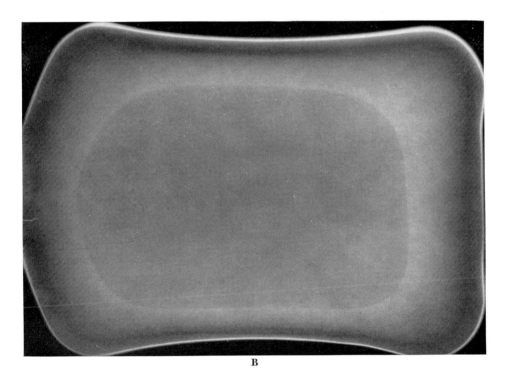

B

FIGURE 3.27.   ILLUSTRATION OF THE DOME SIGN.

A, Lateral projection. This ordinary hot water bottle contains approximately three-fourths water and one-fourth air. In the lateral projection, the dome of air is seen over the fluid within the bag. *B,* Anteroposterior projection, "patient supine." In the anteroposterior projection, the pocket of gas is superimposed on the fluid. A sharp line is seen at the interface between the gas and fluid.

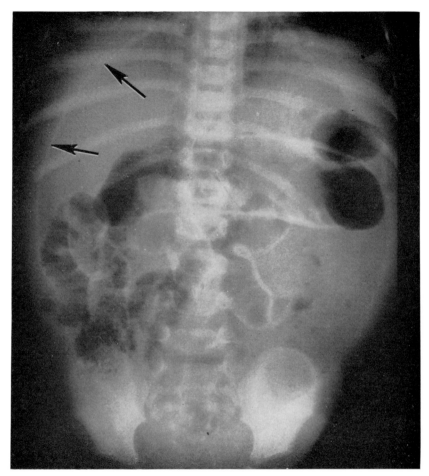

FIGURE 3.28. DOME OR FOOTBALL SIGN; BATTERED CHILD WITH RUPTURED STOMACH.

T.P. This child was in a semicomatose condition with multiple old and new contusions. The abdomen contains air and fluid. When the patient is supine, air forms a dome over the fluid and an interface is formed between the air and fluid (arrows). Large rents in the anterior and posterior wall of the child's stomach were the result of abuse by foster parents.

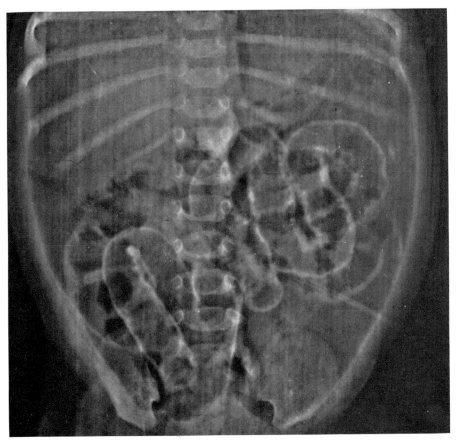

**FIGURE 3.29. VISUALIZATION OF OUTER WALL OF BOWEL; MASSIVE
PNEUMOPERITONEUM FROM GASTRIC RUPTURE; BATTERED CHILD.**

D.M.A., a 3½-months-old white girl, was admitted in a semicomatose condition.
Free air against the outer wall of the small bowel is seen adjacent to the liver.
Gastric rupture is usually accompanied by massive pneumoperitoneum.
(Courtesy of Herbert Abrams, M.D., Stanford University Hospital, Palo Alto,
California.)

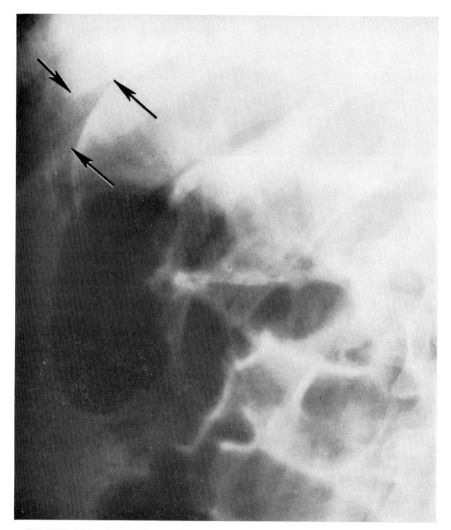

**FIGURE 3.30. AIR ON OUTSIDE OF BOWEL WALL DEMONSTRATED AT
UNDERSURFACE OF LIVER.**

J.McG. had a perforation of the jejunum. Free air on the outside of the bowel
wall is best shown where the bowel lies adjacent to the undersurface of the liver
(arrows).

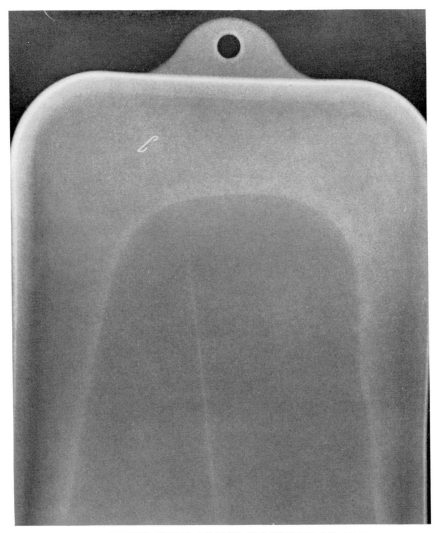

FIGURE 3.31. ILLUSTRATION OF THE FALCIFORM LIGAMENT SIGN.

A hot water bottle was filled with two-thirds water and one-third air. A segment of clear x-ray film was placed within the bag so that the thin edge was parallel to the x-ray beam. On the radiograph it is seen as a thin white line because less dense air is present on both sides of it. With the bottle completely filled with water, the segment of x-ray film is not seen.

attachment of the ligament extends caudally slightly to the right of the midline. Radiographically, when air is present on both sides, the falciform ligament appears as a thin white line (Figs. 9.1 and 3.31). If the patient is rotated, it may be superimposed on the lumbar spine.

REFERENCES

1. Baxter, C. F., and Williams, R. D.: Blunt abdominal trauma. J. Trauma, *1*:241-247, 1961.
2. Blount, R. F., and Lachman, E.: The digestive system. *In* Schaeffer (ed.): Morris' Human Anatomy. 11th ed. New York, Blakiston Division, McGraw Hill Book Co., 1942, p. 1407.
3. Firman-Dahl, J.: Roentgen Examination in Acute Abdominal Diseases. 2nd ed. Springfield, Ill., Charles C Thomas, 1960.
4. Jacobson, G., and Carter, R. A.: Small intestinal rupture due to non-penetrating abdominal injury. Amer. J. Roentgenol., *66*:64-69, 1951.
5. Laurell, H.: A contribution to roentgenological differential diagnosis in the presence of free fluid in the abdomen. Acta Radiol., *16*:424-425, 1935.
6. McCort, J. J.: Rupture or laceration of the liver by non-penetrating trauma. Radiology, *78*:49-57, 1962.
7. Mokrohisky, J.: Pseudopneumoperitoneum. Amer. J. Roentgenol., *79*:293-300, 1958.
8. Williams, R. D., and Zollinger, R. M.: Diagnostic and prognostic factors in abdominal trauma. Amer. J. Surg., *97*:575-578, 1959.

4

SPECIAL RADIOGRAPHIC PROCEDURES: INDICATIONS, TECHNIQUES AND INTERPRETATION

If the extent of visceral injury is not clear on the plain film examination, the radiologist can employ special diagnostic procedures. With experience, these are performed rapidly and interpreted readily. Although the time required for the radiographic examination is increased, these procedures contribute valuable information. In general, a contrast substance is used to outline the suspected organ or to determine the integrity of its vessels.

UPPER GASTROINTESTINAL AND SMALL BOWEL STUDY

Indications

If the patient vomits blood or has blood in his gastric aspirate, laceration of the esophagus, stomach or proximal small bowel is possible and is evaluated by upper gastrointestinal study. With an abnormal position of the diaphragm it is used to rule out a diaphragmatic tear with visceral herniation. It is not necessary when free intraperitoneal air is present.

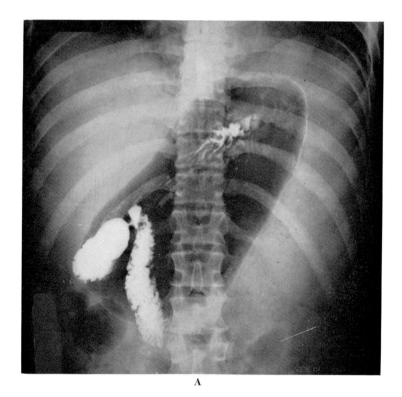

A

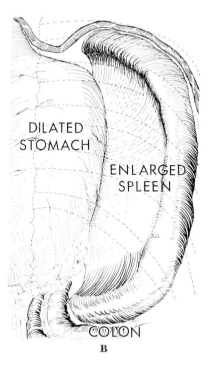

B

Figure 4.1.   *See legend on opposite page.*

Technique

A water-soluble radiopaque medium such as 25 per cent diatrizoate sodium* or diatrizoate methylglucamine† is administered orally or by naso-gastric tube. If perforation is present, the diatrizoate leaks into the peri-toneal cavity, from which it is readily absorbed.

Interpretation

In the presence of perforation of the stomach or small bowel, the water-soluble opaque material enters the peritoneal cavity.

Intramural hematoma appears as a filling defect in the intestinal lumen. The mucosal folds are flattened and thickened when the hemorrhage and edema involve the submucosal layer. With extensive hemorrhage, the lumen is obstructed.

Opacification of the upper gastrointestinal tract also gives information about adjacent viscera. Perisplenic hematoma displaces the stomach and small bowel downward and to the right. A tear in the diaphragm permits herniation of the stomach or small bowel into the thorax. Failure of the opaque medium to pass into a herniated stomach or small bowel indicates incarceration.

COLON EXAMINATION

Indications

(1) Blood found at the rectal orifice or on digital examination suggests laceration of the colon. If free air is present in the peritoneal cavity, no further examination need be carried out as immediate surgery is indicated. (2) In suspected hemoperitoneum the colon is identified with certainty when outlined by plain air enema (Fig. 4.2A and B).

---

* Diatrizoate sodium: Hypaque, Winthrop Laboratories.
† Diatrizoate methylglucamine: Renografin, E. R. Squibb and Sons.

(Illustration on opposite page.)

FIGURE 4.1. BARIUM SWALLOW TO SHOW STOMACH DISPLACEMENT BY SPLENIC MASS.

A, Plain film. E.L. Enlargement of the spleen causes medial displacement of barium-and-gas-filled stomach and downward displacement of the splenic flexure. B, Diagram.
(Courtesy of John von Saltza, M.D., San Jose Hospital, San Jose, California.)

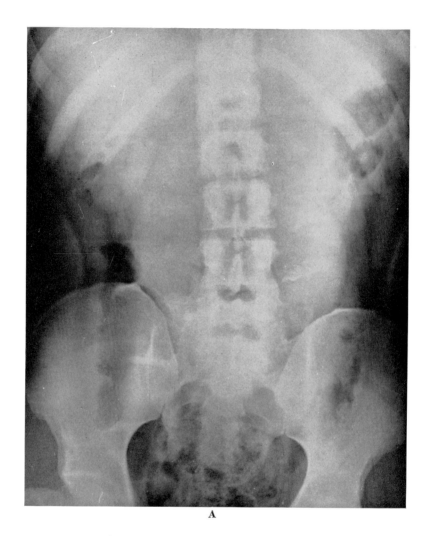

A

Figure 4.2. *See legend on opposite page.*

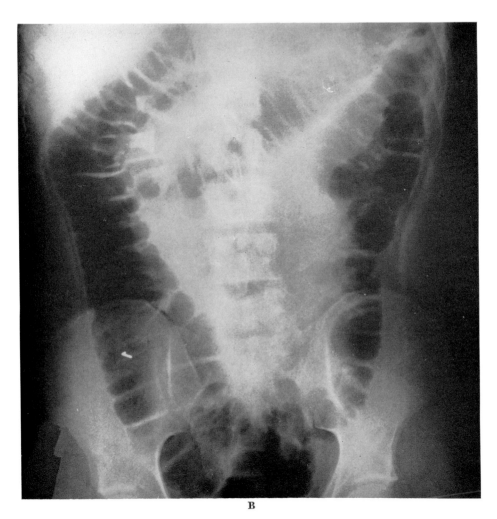

B

FIGURE 4.2.   AIR ENEMA TO RULE OUT INTRAPERITONEAL BLEEDING.

A, Preliminary. C.P. The initial radiographic examination revealed fractures of the left transverse processes of L2 to L5 with retroperitoneal hematoma. An increased space between the ascending colon and the properitoneal fat on the right suggested bleeding. *B,* Air enema. The inflated ascending colon is adjacent to the properitoneal fat, excluding the likelihood of intraperitoneal bleeding.

Technique

(1) To detect perforation, the colon is examined by means of an enema of 20 to 40 per cent diatrizoate sodium.[10]   (2) To show the position of the colon in relation to the extraperitoneal fat, a quantity of air sufficient to distend the colon is administered rectally.

Interpretation

The escape of the contrast material into the peritoneum identifies a perforation of the colon or terminal ileum (Fig. 9.16).

PNEUMOPERITONEOGRAPHY

Indications

This examination is used to outline the liver, spleen or pelvic organs. It can be accomplished as part of a four quadrant diagnostic tap.

Technique

After the abdomen is inspected to assure the absence of surgical scars, which would indicate adhesions, a site is selected in either the left upper or lower quadrant (any site may be utilized) and prepared with an anti-septic. A local skin anesthetic wheal is raised and the peritoneum is punctured with a 6-inch No. 18 or 20 needle. A short bevel on the needle is desirable. It is directed medially to avoid pinning a viscus against the curved posterior abdominal wall. With the needle in the peritoneal space, gas is delivered by a controlled metered system. The injection is painless. An extraperitoneal injection is indicated when there is crepitation of the subcutaneous tissues or asymmetric filling of the abdomen. The escape of gas around the needle or absence of a tympanitic percussion note on the opposite side also indicates a faulty position of the needle. When this occurs, the needle is repositioned. One thousand to 1500 milliliters are injected.[11]

The ideal gas for this examination is carbon dioxide, as it is a normal constituent of the blood and is quickly absorbed from the peritoneal cavity. Because of the rapid absorption, the radiographic examination must follow promptly. Nitrous oxide is also utilized; being less soluble than carbon dioxide, it remains in the peritoneal cavity longer.

The radiographic exposure time is reduced by half to allow for pneumatization of the abdomen. Simultaneous pneumatization and visceral opacification studies are sometimes advantageous.

Interpretation

By placing the patient in prone, lateral decubitus, and upright positions a three-dimensional view of the surface of the liver or spleen is obtained (Fig. 4.3). An abnormal protuberance on the surface of these organs suggests subcapsular hematoma[1] (Fig. 6.3). Failure of gas to dissect between the organ and the peritoneal surface indicates adhesions, from either injury or infection. Free blood in the peritoneal cavity will appear as a fluid level on films taken with a horizontal beam (Fig. 4.4).

Both carbon dioxide and nitrous oxide are readily absorbed from the peritoneal surface. If the patient is uncomfortable following this examination, the needle is re-inserted and the gas allowed to escape.

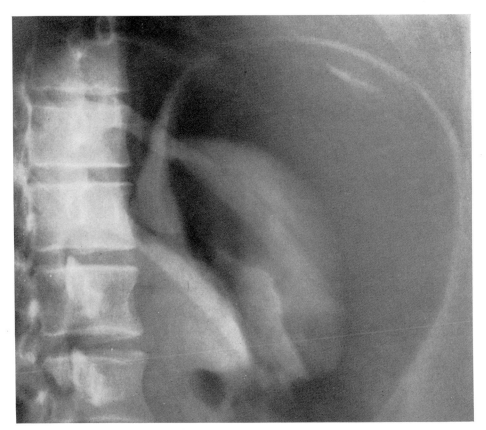

FIGURE 4.3. PNEUMOPERITONEOGRAPHY; NORMAL SPLEEN.

A rupture of the spleen was suspected in this patient, but the plain film of the abdomen was within normal limits. This diagnostic pneumoperitoneum shows a smooth spleen and no evidence of blood in the peritoneal cavity.

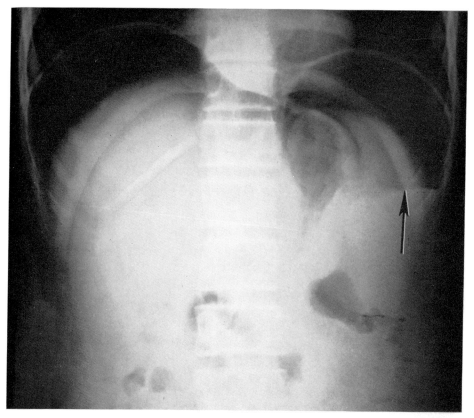

FIGURE 4.4. PNEUMOPERITONEOGRAPHY; INTRAPERITONEAL BLOOD.

D.C. had been kicked in the abdomen by a horse (see Fig. 2.2). The plain film of the abdomen showed splenic enlargement and fluid in the left flank. Nitrous oxide, 1200 milliliters, was introduced into the peritoneal cavity. The enlargement of the spleen is confirmed, and there is a level of free blood within the peritoneal cavity (arrow).

ARTERIOGRAPHY

Indications

Trauma to the abdominal viscera results in vessel contusion or transection. Arteriography uniquely demonstrates the extent of vascular damage. It is most valuable when the bleeding is subcapsular or intraparenchymal. Visualization of the arterial tree is obtained either by selective catheterization or retrograde brachial injection.

Technique

FEMORAL ARTERY CATHETERIZATION. The skin of the groin is shaved and washed. An area of skin over the femoral pulsation just distal to the inguinal ligament is infiltrated with anesthetic. A small skin incision is made in the anesthetized area and the tissues down to the femoral artery are spread by a small hemostat. A Seldinger No. 160 needle is inserted until the pulse can be detected through the top of the needle. The needle is then thrust through the artery, transfixing it (Fig. 4.5). The sharp stylet is removed. The outer needle is depressed and slowly withdrawn. When the needle is well centered in the artery, blood will spurt from the open end. The metal guide wire is held in readiness by the assistant and the flexible tip is quickly inserted through the needle. The guide wire is advanced several inches into the artery and then the needle is withdrawn from the artery over the guide wire. Digital pressure on the artery is maintained while the guide wire alone is in the artery.[9]

A preformed radiopaque catheter is inserted into the vessel over the guide wire. Under fluoroscopic or television observation, the tip of the catheter is advanced up the aorta to a point opposite the origin of the selected vessel. The guide wire is pulled back from the tip of the catheter. With the proper curvature given to the tip, the catheter is introduced directly into the arterial branch (selective arteriography) (Fig. 4.6). By repeated aspiration is is ascertained that the catheter does not occlude the artery. An injection of 8 to 10 milliliters of 50 per cent diatrizoate is made (Fig. 4.7).

AXILLARY ARTERY CATHETERIZATION. Selective arteriography can be done by axillary artery catheterization if the femoral vessels are not suitable.[2, 5, 7, 8] With the patient's left arm abducted to 90°, the axilla is shaved; antiseptic is applied to the skin, and the tissues over the artery are anesthetized with 1 or 2 per cent Xylocaine. The technique of Seldinger,[9] outlined in the preceding paragraph, is employed. Under fluoroscopic control the tip of the catheter is advanced down the thoracic aorta. After the guide wire is withdrawn from the tip of the catheter, the catheter is inserted in the selected branch of the abdominal aorta (Fig. 4.6).

At this point, the guide wire is removed and 10 milliliters of diatrizoate is injected manually. Films of the opacified artery and its branches are taken with a rapid cassette changer.

RETROGRADE BRACHIAL INJECTION. An alternative method of studying the abdominal viscera is by the percutaneous injection of opaque material into the left brachial artery. A Seldinger No. 160 or Karras needle is inserted percutaneously. With a pressure of 450 pounds per square inch, 100 milliliters of 50 per cent diatrizoate is injected. The opaque material passes in a retrograde fashion into the descending thoracic aorta and then outlines the abdominal aorta and its major branches.[4] Since all the abdominal vessels are perfused simultaneously, this method is not as precise as the selective femoral or axillary technique, but it requires far less time.

TECHNIQUE OF INTRODUCING CATHETER INTO FEMORAL OR AXILLARY ARTERY

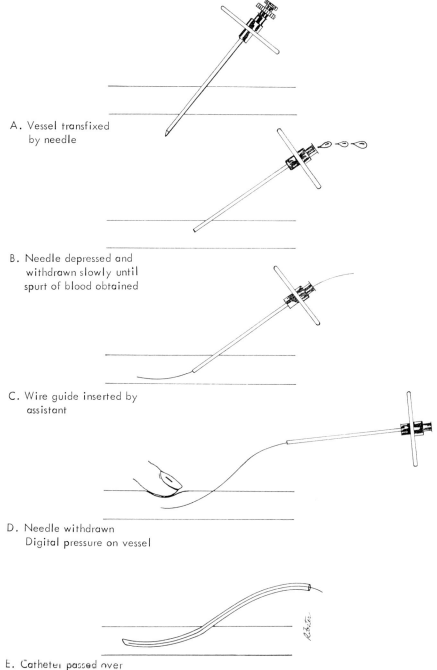

A. Vessel transfixed
   by needle

B. Needle depressed and
   withdrawn slowly until
   spurt of blood obtained

C. Wire guide inserted by
   assistant

D. Needle withdrawn
   Digital pressure on vessel

E. Catheter passed over
   guide wire

**FIGURE 4.5. DIAGRAM: SELDINGER TECHNIQUE FOR SELECTIVE
ARTERIOGRAPHY.[9]**

INTRODUCTION OF CATHETER INTO CELIAC AXIS

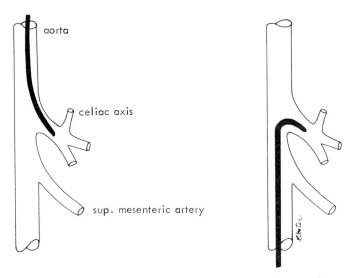

A. Axillary approach
down thoracic aorta

B. Femoral approach
up abdominal aorta

FIGURE 4.6. DIAGRAM: SELECTIVE CATHETERIZATION OF THE CELIAC AXIS.

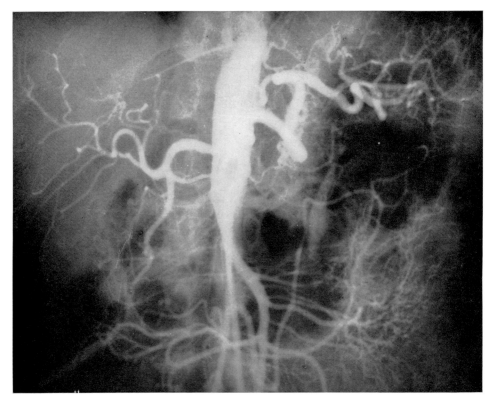

**FIGURE 4.7. SELECTIVE ARTERIOGRAPHY; NORMAL CELIAC AXIS AND
SUPERIOR MESENTERIC ARTERY.**

R.V., a 47-year-old woman, was examined for persistent abdominal pain. By
means of the Seldinger technique, a catheter was introduced through the right
femoral artery into the celiac axis. Another was passed through the left femoral
artery into the superior mesenteric artery. Simultaneous opacification of these
vessels shows their normal appearance. This examination is valuable in the
study of suspected trauma to the liver, spleen and pancreas.

Interpretation

A displacement of the arteries within the viscus with pooling of the
opaque medium indicates subcapsular or parenchymal hematoma (Fig.
4.8*A* and *B*). Extravasation of opaque material points to continuous free
bleeding. Areas of avascularity due to vessel occlusion are shown by this
method.

The study of the arterial tree is particularly important in injury to
the kidneys.

RADIOACTIVE ISOTOPE SCANNING

In essence, these techniques demonstrate a loss of blood supply to an
organ. Scanning has been used to delineate vascular injury in both the
liver and kidneys.

Liver Scan

Indications

Central necrosis from intraparenchymal tears of the liver is demonstrated by this examination.

Technique

Colloidal AU[198], 1.5 microcuries per kilogram of body weight, is in jected intravenously, with a maximum dose of 100 μc. The isotope is deposited in the reticuloendothelial cells and the scan can be done from 1 to 48 hours after injection. At this level of activity, the radiation dose to the liver is approximately 5 rads.

Rose bengal tagged with I[131] (2.5 to 3.0 μc. per kg.) is picked up and excreted by the polygonal cells of the liver. Scanning is done 30 minutes after the injection.

The patient is placed in a supine position with the probe as close as possible to the skin. Both the liver and spleen are included in the scan. The xyphoid and right lower rib margin are noted as landmarks. Routinely the liver is scanned in anteroposterior and lateral projections (Fig. 4.9).

Interpretation

An area of low activity indicates necrosis of the liver cells from intraparenchymal tearing (Fig. 7.5).

Kidney Scan

Indications

When the injured kidney does not excrete diatrizoate or when visualization of the kidneys is poor for technical reasons, renal scanning is used. It is particularly valuable for use with a patient who has an allergy to iodide.

Technique

Chlormerodrin tagged with Hg[197] or Hg[203] is given intravenously. Hg[197] has a physical half life of 2.7 days and an energy of 77 KEV. The adult dose is 125 to 150 microcuries.[3, 6] Hg[203] has a physical half life of 48 days and an energy of 279 KEV. The adult dose is 100 microcuries. With Hg[197] radiation to the kidney is one-tenth that of Hg[203]. Scans are made with the patient prone and are started one hour after administration of the isotope.

Interpretation

An area of low activity in the kidney signifies vascular damage.

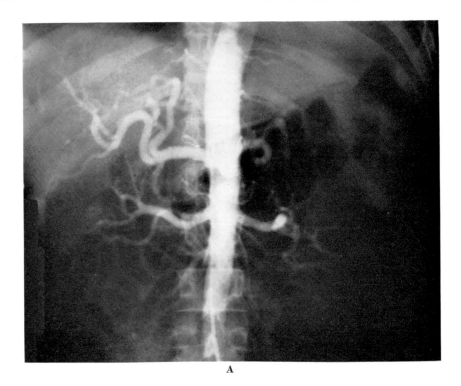

A

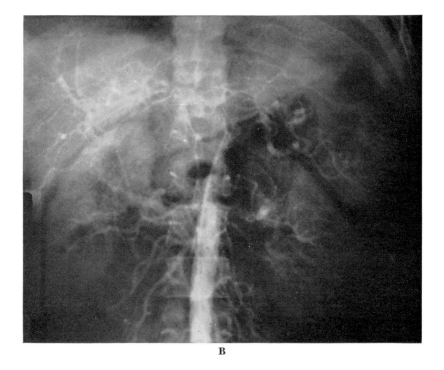

B

Figure 4.8 A and B. *4.8 C and legend on following page.*

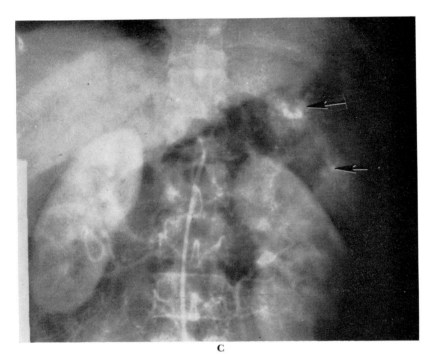

C

**FIGURE 4.8. CENTRAL LACERATION OF THE SPLEEN DEMONSTRATED
BY ARTERIOGRAPHY.**

A, Early arterial phase. *B,* Late arterial phase. *C,* Capillary phase. R.S. after
an accident, developed abdominal and left shoulder pain. The hematocrit was
within normal limits. He had a fracture of the left 12th rib posteriorly, associated with left hemothorax and obscuration of the left leaf of the diaphragm.
Retrograde femoral arteriography shows extravasation of the diatrizoate within
two areas of the spleen, indicating intraparenchymal bleeding (arrows). The
splenic outline is intact.

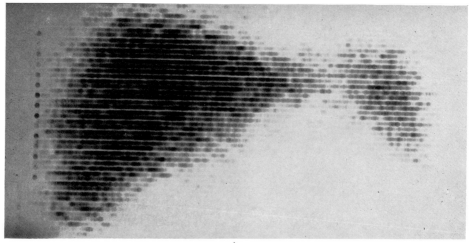

A

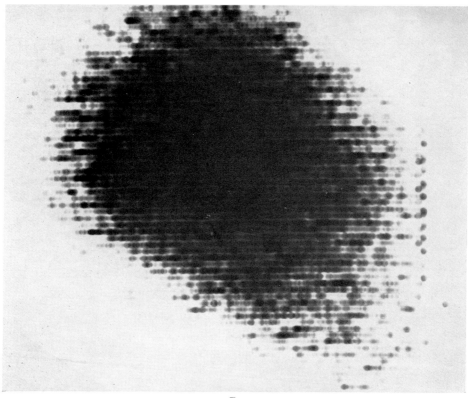

B

**FIGURE 4.9. NORMAL RADIOACTIVE SCINTILLATION SCAN OF
LIVER AND SPLEEN.**

A, Anteroposterior. D.M. was given 150 μc. of radioactive gold intravenously.
The scan was obtained at 24 hours; both liver and spleen are well shown. A
notch on the undersurface of the liver represents the gallbladder fossa. *B,* Right
lateral projection. The liver is sharply outlined and the anterior border is lower
than the posterior.

UROGRAPHY

Indications

Hematuria is the prime sign of urinary tract injury, and the initial diagnostic study is intravenous urography. Contusion of the flanks, fractures of the lower posterior ribs and fractures of the transverse processes of the lumbar spine suggest possible renal or ureteral damage.

Technique

Thirty milliliters of 50 per cent diatrizoate sodium or 60 per cent diatrizoate methylglucamine are injected intravenously and films are obtained at intervals of five minutes. Since these patients are unprepared for the examination, visualization may be poor. After 15 minutes, if the urinary tract is not adequately seen, an additional 30 milliliters of diatrizoate are given.

Interpretation

As the spectrum of renal injuries ranges from mild contusion to complete fragmentation, a variety of changes may be encountered on the intravenous urogram. Interference with the blood supply or the excretory function will result in nonvisualization. This is prima-facie evidence of injury but it does not adequately define its extent. If the collecting structures are visualized, irregularity of the calyceal and pelvic outlines indicates parenchymal tears. Extravasation is a rare finding, occurring when one pole of the kidney is torn while the uninjured fragment continues to excrete the dye. Blood clots in the calyces, pelvis, ureters or bladder cast negative shadows within these dye-filled structures.

CYSTOGRAPHY

Indications

Compression injuries to the lower abdomen and fractures of the pelvis with hematuria suggest bladder trauma. The cystogram obtained following intravenous urography may show this. In the doubtful case, direct cystographic examination is performed.

Technique

A sterile Foley catheter is inserted transurethrally and 100 to 200 milliliters of 25 per cent solution of sterile, water-soluble iodide are injected into the bladder. Films are taken in the anteroposterior, oblique and lateral projections. Radiographs with cephalad and caudad 30° angulation of the tube will improve the delineation of the bladder wall.

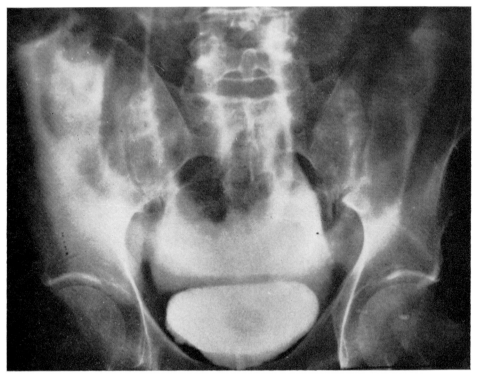

FIGURE 4.10. CYSTOGRAPHIC EXAMINATION OF THE BLADDER.

To evaluate a suspected tear, 200 milliliters of opaque medium are injected into the bladder through a Foley catheter. In this injured patient, the radiopaque solution escaped into the peritoneal cavity. This radiopaque fluid above the bladder simulates the projecting ears of a dog—the "dog's ears sign."
(Courtesy of William Marshall, M.D., Stanford University Hospital, Palo Alto, California.)

Interpretation

Intraperitoneal or retroperitoneal extravasation is shown when the opaque material appears outside the bladder (Fig. 4.10). An irregularity of the bladder wall is a sign of contusion with submucosal hemorrhage.

URETHROGRAPHY

Indications

This examination is done when there has been a perineal injury and when the patient is unable to void or cannot be catheterized.

Technique

Under sterile conditions, a 25 per cent solution of water-soluble iodide is introduced into the urethra through a Brodny catheter. Right and left oblique films show the course of the urethra.

Interpretation

Extravasation may occur above the urogenital diaphragm into the retroperitoneal tissues or below the diaphragm into the perineal and scrotal tissues.

REFERENCES

1. Birsner, J. W., Wallner, A., and Leask, M. D.: Roentgen diagnosis of rupture of the spleen by pneumoperitoneum. J. Int. Coll. Surg., *20*:338-342, 1953.
2. Hanafee, W.: Axillary artery approach to carotid, vertebral, abdominal aorta, and coronary angiography. Radiology, *81*:559-567, 1963.
3. Izenstark, J. L., Burden, J. J., Mardis, H. K., and Varella, R.: Clinical indications for kidney scanning. J.A.M.A., *136*:128-139, 1964.
4. Marshall, T. R., Ling, J. T., and Gonzalez, R.: Additional experiences with direct percutaneous noncatheter brachial angiography — left panarteriography — right cerebral angiography. Radiology, *81*:568-575, 1963.
5. Newton, T. H.: The axillary artery approach to arteriography of the aorta and its branches. Amer. J. Roentgenol., *89*:275-283, 1963.
6. Quinn, J. L., and Maynard, C. D.: Renal radioisotope scintiscanning. Radiol. Clin. North America, *3*:65-74, 1965.
7. Riley, J. M., Hanafee, W., and Weidner, W.: Left axillary approach to the abdominal aorta. Radiology, *84*:96-99, 1965.
8. Roy, P.: Percutaneous catheterization via the axillary artery. Amer. J. Roentgenol., *94*:1-18, 1965.
9. Seldinger, S. I.: Catheter replacement of needle in percutaneous arteriography. New technique. Acta Radiol., *39*:368-376, 1953.
10. Shehadi, W. H.: Studies of the colon and small intestine with water-soluble iodinated contrast material. Amer. J. Roentgenol., *89*:740-751, 1963.
11. Stevens, G. M., and McCort, J. J.: Abdominal pneumoperitoneography. Radiology, *83*:480-485, 1964.

5

PHENOMENON OF DELAYED RUPTURE AND BLEEDING

CLINICAL OBSERVATIONS

Delayed rupture and bleeding is a feature of blunt abdominal trauma and this possibility must be kept in mind for proper management of the injured person.

In the typical case, the results of radiographic examination on admission may be within normal limits. Shortly thereafter, the vital signs stabilize and symptoms subside. After an interval that may vary from hours to weeks, there is a recurrence of symptoms and clinical signs of bleeding. At this point, an immediate repeat radiographic examination, including special procedures, is useful. Radiographic signs of rupture and bleeding may then be apparent on comparison with the initial films.

THEORETICAL CONSIDERATIONS

The mechanism by which delayed rupture and bleeding occurs is not definitely known. Zabrinski and Harkins[5] discuss eight different theories which have been advanced to explain delayed rupture of the spleen. Two of the most plausible theories are as follows:

1. Hematoma breakdown. The initial injury causes a subcapsular or subserosal hematoma. With continued oozing into the contused tissues,

the hematoma breaks down, spilling a large quantity of blood into the peritoneal or retroperitoneal space. With the muscular viscera (such as the diaphragm, the bowel or the bladder), contusion of a portion of the muscle may cause necrosis. Later, the necrotic segment gives way, leading to extrusion of the contents or, when the diaphragm is involved, herniation of abdominal viscera into the thorax.

2. Delayed clot detachment. According to this theory, the initial injury produces a tear and bleeding. A clot forms over the tear and repair begins. Later, because of movement of the organ or increase in blood pressure, the clot is detached and bleeding resumes.

FREQUENCY

The experience of the Santa Clara County Hospital and Medical Center with delayed rupture is shown in Table 5.1. In one patient, a rent in the left leaf of the diaphragm became clinically manifest by shock and dyspnea 37 days after injury. Delayed rupture of the spleen was documented in five patients, the longest interval being eight days after injury. Donhauser and Locke,[2] in their analysis of 68 cases of splenic rupture, found that a delay occurred in 28 per cent. Interestingly, the mortality was only one-half that in cases of immediate rupture.

In a review of reported cases of splenic rupture up to 1956, Bollinger and Fowler[1] found that 21.5 per cent had delayed perforation. This incidence seems high; it is possible that some cases represent delayed diagnosis rather than perforation.

A patient with delayed rupture of the liver and another with delayed rupture of the colon were seen. A delayed infarction of the ileum has been reported by Hughes and Smaill[4] and by Duncan.[3]

Even though the patient's clinical condition apparently returns to normal after the injury, delayed rupture can occur. Careful repeated clinical and radiographic examinations will help detect delayed ruptures and perforations. When the patient leaves the hospital, he must be warned to report any sudden change in his condition.

Table 5.1. Delayed Rupture

ORGAN	NO. OF CASES	INTERVAL
Spleen	5	5 to 8 days
Liver	1	7 days
Diaphragm	5	2 to 37 days
Colon	2	10 to 15 days
Kidney	1	60 days

REFERENCES

1. Bollinger, J. A., and Fowler, E. F.: Traumatic rupture of the spleen with special
   reference to delayed splenic rupture. Amer. J. Surg., *91*:561-570, 1956.
2. Donhauser, J. L., and Locke, D. J.: Traumatic rupture of the spleen. An analysis of
   sixty-eight cases. A.M.A. Arch. Surg., *80*:153-158, 1960.
3. Duncan, J. T.: Rupture of the small intestine through the intact abdominal wall
   without associated intraperitoneal injury. Amer. Surgeon, *22*:1215-1221, 1956.
4. Hughes, L. E., and Smaill, G. B.: Long-delayed complications of closed abdominal
   trauma. Brit. Med. J., *1*:776-777, 1962.
5. Zabrinski, E. J., and Harkins, H. N.: Delayed splenic rupture: A clinical syndrome
   following trauma. Report of 4 cases with an analysis of 177 cases collected from
   the literature. Arch. Surg., *46*:186-213, 1943.

6

LACERATION OF THE SPLEEN

CLINICAL OBSERVATIONS

Because it is the intraperitoneal organ most frequently injured, the spleen is always carefully studied. Persistent severe left upper quadrant pain aggravated by breathing or lying in the supine position suggests splenic injury. Left shoulder pain is a prominent symptom. The patient may complain of a sense of fullness in the left upper quadrant. In some cases, leukocytosis is found.

The spleen abnormally enlarged by disease is more easily ruptured. Cases have been reported in which rupture followed very mild trauma, even palpation by an examining physician. Conditions which render the spleen more liable to tear include malaria, infectious mononucleosis, congestive splenomegaly, sarcoidosis and Gaucher's disease. Pregnancy is thought to increase the likelihood of splenic rupture in abdominal trauma.[15]

A small rupture with subcapsular hematoma may not be recognized at the time of injury. At a later date the patient may present with a left upper quadrant mass and an anemia simulating a blood dyscrasia or neoplasm (Fig. 6.1).[8]

ASSOCIATED INJURIES

The most common associated injury is fracture of the left lower ribs with contusion of the soft tissues of the upper abdominal wall. In the

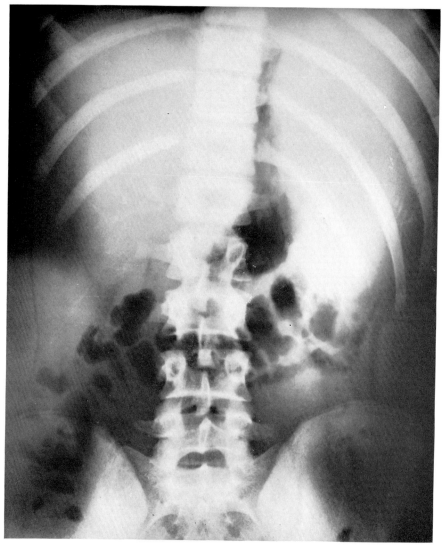

FIGURE 6.1. SPLENOMEGALY DUE TO UNSUSPECTED SUBCAPSULAR HEMATOMA;
SIMULATION OF LYMPHOMA.

R.C. had upper abdominal pain, hemoglobin-deficient microcytic anemia and a microscopic hematuria suggesting a blood dyscrasia or lymphoma. On the radiograph, a splenic mass compresses the stomach and displaces it medially. At operation, an enlarged hemorrhagic spleen was adherent to the diaphragm, kidney and mesentery. The boy had played football two weeks before, but had no memory of injury.
(Courtesy of George Magid, M.D., San Jose, California.)

author's series, fractures of the left lower ribs were found in 20 of 51 cases of splenic injury.

Maughon et al.[9] report a 21 per cent incidence of rupture of the left hemidiaphragm associated with injuries of the spleen. Next in order of frequency is contusion or rupture of the left kidney. In the study of Shirkey et al.[14] the mortality was directly proportional to the number of associated injuries. More than half of all deaths resulted from hemorrhage.

RADIOGRAPHIC EXAMINATION

Plain Film Examination

The outline of the spleen can be seen only in about 60 per cent of abdominal radiographs.[19] The finding of a small, sharply defined and normally shaped spleen in the left upper quadrant is good but not conclusive evidence that the spleen is intact.[18]

In uncomplicated injury of the spleen, the left kidney and left psoas muscle outlines remain visible (Fig. 6.7). Hemorrhage from splenic injury is almost always intraperitoneal and the fat which surrounds the kidney and psoas is undisturbed. If the kidney and psoas are obscured on the left in comparison with the right, concomitant retroperitoneal injury is likely.[4]

Opacification of the Stomach or Splenic Flexure of the Colon

The approximate size of the spleen can be evaluated when the splenic flexure of the colon and the stomach are outlined by gas. In the doubtful case, air or barium is introduced into the stomach and splenic flexure of the colon (Fig. 6.2).

Chest Film and Fluoroscopy

Injury to the spleen is accompanied frequently by a contusion or rupture of the diaphragm. Hemorrhage beneath the diaphragm causes muscle splinting. As a result, excursion of the diaphragm is reduced. Serial films of the chest and fluoroscopy show elevation of the diaphragm or limitation of its motion.[2]

Pneumoperitoneography

If the spleen cannot be visualized on the plain film, subcapsular or intraparenchymal bleeding is evaluated by pneumoperitoneography. Films are taken in the upright, prone and right lateral decubitus projections. A

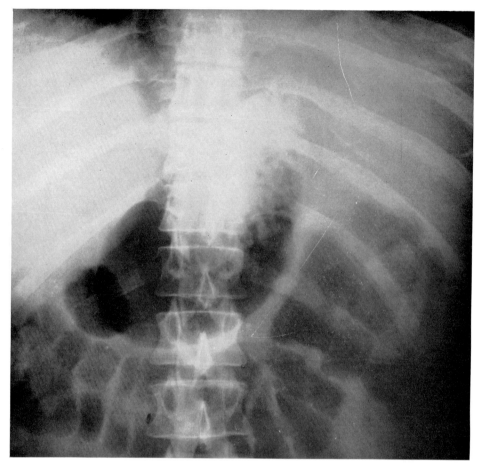

FIGURE 6.2. MEDIAL DISPLACEMENT OF THE STOMACH BY SPLENIC MASS; DELAYED RUPTURE OF THE SPLEEN (7 DAYS).

P.R. had sustained an abdominal injury one week prior to hospital admission. On entry he had left upper quadrant pain and rapidly went into shock. A large mass in the left upper quadrant displaces the diatrizoate-filled stomach toward the midline and the splenic flexure downward. At operation, the mass consisted of splenic fragments and hemorrhage.

normal splenic outline makes a subcapsular hematoma unlikely. A bulge in the surface of the spleen is evidence of a subcapsular hematoma (Fig. 6.3). Adherence of the spleen to the undersurface of the diaphragm or to the lateral abdominal wall results from injury or infection.

Splenic Arteriography

This is performed by femoral or axillary catheterization, or by retrograde brachial injection. Opaque medium is injected into the celiac axis while rapid filming is done.[10] Pooling of the opaque medium in the

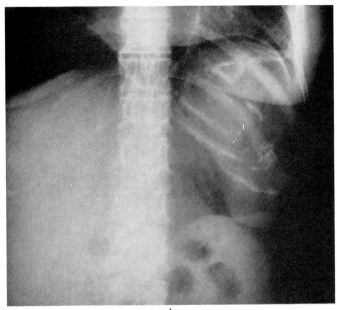

A

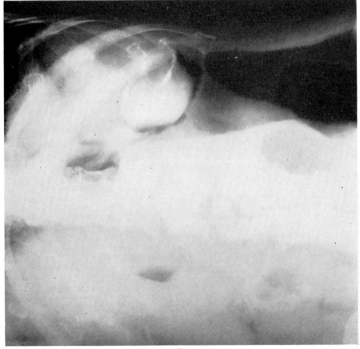

B

FIGURE 6.3. SUBCAPSULAR HEMATOMA OF SPLEEN; PNEUMOPERITONEOGRAPHY.

A, Upright film. A.R. Two weeks prior to admission this woman had been struck in the abdomen. Splenic enlargement was found on the plain films. Pneumoperitoneography shows a bulbous enlargement of the lower pole of the spleen and the upper pole adherent to the undersurface of the diaphragm. *B,* Right lateral decubitus film. At operation, an old tear in the capsule of the upper pole with adhesions to the diaphragm was found. A subcapsular hematoma caused the bulbous enlargement of the lower pole.

79

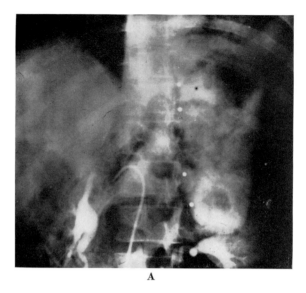

A

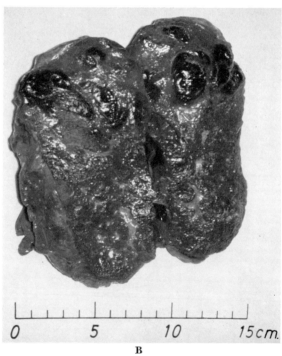

B

Figure 6.4. *See legend on opposite page.*

subcapsular or the intraparenchymal portion of the spleen indicates hemorrhage (Fig. 6.4).

TYPES OF SPLENIC BLEEDING

Radiographically, three types of bleeding are encountered: (1) subcapsular hematoma, (2) splenic fossa hemorrhage, and (3) free intraperitoneal bleeding. In some patients, all three are found.

Subcapsular Hematoma

This results from a tear in the splenic pulp with hematoma formation beneath an intact capsule and is relatively infrequent. In 51 cases of splenic injury seen at the Santa Clara County Hospital, only three patients had a subcapsular hematoma alone. Hemorrhage beneath the capsule will cause a bulge of a portion of the spleen, or the entire spleen may enlarge, displacing the stomach and splenic flexure of the colon. Subcapsular hematoma is well shown by pneumoperitoneography (Fig. 6.3) or arteriography (Fig. 6.4).

Subcapsular hematoma is an indication for splenectomy. If the patient refuses operative treatment, he is warned that he may have subsequent bleeding episodes.

An untreated splenic hematoma either is absorbed or undergoes liquefaction to form a splenic pseudocyst (Fig. 6.5). Splenic pseudocysts with secondary mural calcification have been reported.[6, 12] Next to parasitic infection, trauma is the most common cause of splenic cyst.[11] In children, splenic cyst is almost always the result of trauma.

Hemorrhage into the Splenic Fossa

This follows a localized extravasation of blood. It was found only in 2 of 51 cases studied. The hemorrhagic mass in the left upper quadrant

---

(Illustration on opposite page.)

**FIGURE 6.4. INTRAPARENCHYMAL BLEEDING OF THE SPLEEN;
SELECTIVE ARTERIOGRAPHY.**

A, Selective arteriogram, late venous phase. R.J. sustained an injury to the left upper quadrant and a mass developed in the region of the spleen. A retrograde femoral arteriogram with the catheter tip in the celiac axis shows pools of contrast medium within the parenchyma of an enlarged spleen. The left kidney is displaced downward. *B,* Specimen. After splenectomy, areas of hemorrhage within the spleen were found.
(Courtesy of Tord Olin, M.D., Lund, Sweden.)

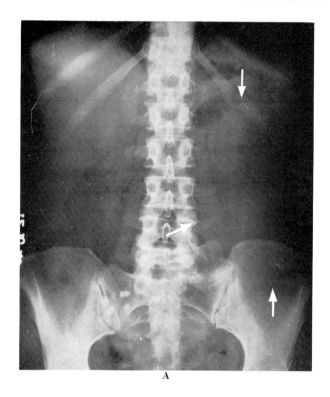

A

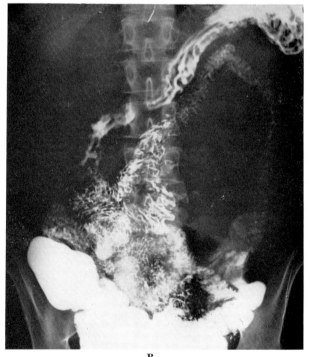

B

Figure 6.5. *See legend on opposite page.*

displaces the stomach medially and the splenic flexure downward, similar to subcapsular hematoma. The normal outline of the spleen is lost. With these findings on the plain film, rupture is indicated, and no further studies are needed (Fig. 6.6). If the findings are equivocal, arteriography is helpful. Extravasation of the injected opaque medium from the spleen is evidence of laceration.[10, 16]

Free Intraperitoneal Bleeding

This is the most common result of splenic laceration and occurred in all but 5 of 51 cases studied. Varying amounts of blood in the flanks and pelvis are accompanied by a left upper quadrant mass consisting of the fragments of the spleen and surrounding hematoma (Figs. 6.7 and 6.8). The splenic mass displaces the stomach and colon away from the splenic fossa.

Gaseous distention of the stomach is seen in splenic injury.[5] This nonspecific finding occurred in 13 of 51 cases. It may result from adynamic ileus due to injury of the stomach aided by air swallowing in an apprehensive patient (Figs. 6.9 and 6.10).

An elevated left leaf of the diaphragm with limited excursion is due either to the accumulation of blood beneath or to a concomitant injury of the diaphragm (Fig. 6.11). Progressive loss of mobility of the left leaf of the diaphragm has been noted by Cimmino,[2] who recommends repeated fluoroscopic examination to detect this valuable sign. Discoid atelectasis at the left lung base may accompany loss of diaphragmatic mobility.

Fluid in the left chest was present in 14 of 51 patients with splenic rupture; usually there were concomitant fractures of the left lower ribs. A patient with infrapulmonary effusion as the major roentgenographic sign of spleen laceration has been reported by Kittredge and Finby.[7]

Serration of the greater curvature side of the stomach has been described as a sign of splenic rupture and is believed to be due to the dissection of the blood into the gastrosplenic ligament.[5] Schwartz et al.[13]

(Illustration on opposite page.)

FIGURE 6.5. TRAUMATIC PSEUDOCYST OF THE SPLEEN.

A, Plain film. M.F. had pain and a rapidly enlarging mass in the left upper abdomen. A known alcoholic with cirrhosis, she had fallen previously, fracturing several ribs. This plain film shows the smooth left upper quadrant mass (arrows). The kidney and psoas margins are intact. *B,* Gastrointestinal series. The left upper quadrant mass displaces the stomach and small bowel to the right. An old traumatic pseudocyst, in which recent hemorrhage had taken place, was removed.

(Courtesy of C. C. Wang, M.D., Massachusetts General Hospital, Boston, Massachusetts.)

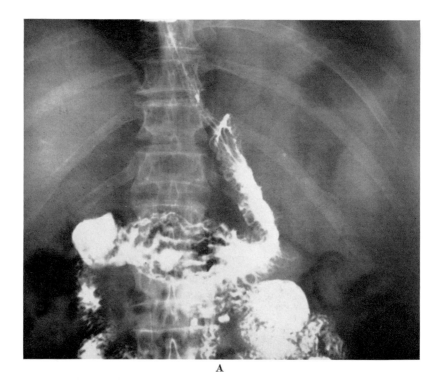

A

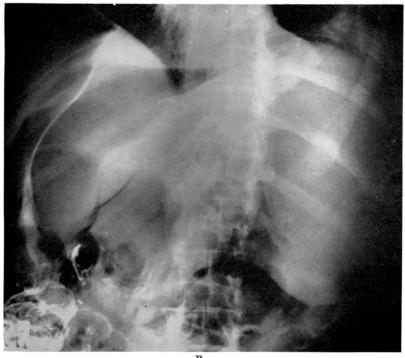

B

Figure 6.6. *See legend on opposite page.*

studied the roentgenograms in 12 children with rupture of the spleen and found exaggerated folds in the greater curvature of the stomach in seven. This was the only roentgen sign occurring with any degree of frequency. At Santa Clara County Hospital, serration of the greater curvature of the stomach was present in only 2 of 51 cases. It is an uncommon finding in splenic injury.

DELAYED RUPTURE OF THE SPLEEN

This has been the subject of several extensive reports (Chapter 5). It may follow a subcapsular hematoma and is the reason why a spleen showing subcapsular hemorrhage should be removed. Delayed rupture is signaled by the onset of left upper quadrant pain and shock (Figs. 6.2 and 6.11). If follow-up radiographs show intraperitoneal bleeding, whereas the initial abdominal film was negative, delayed rupture has occurred.

According to the study of Terry, Self and Howard[17] delayed ruptures of the spleen follow a latent period of less than one week in 50 per cent of patients and less than two weeks in 75 per cent. Zabrinski and Harkins[20] have reported a patient with delayed rupture and hemorrhage two years after the initial trauma. Bollinger and Fowler[1] found that fluid at the left lung base on radiographs taken more than 24 hours after injury is highly suggestive of delayed rupture.

SPLENOSIS

A rare complication of splenic fragmentation is the seeding of peritoneal surfaces. This can occur when all portions of the ruptured spleen are not or cannot be removed at surgery. These implanted spleen fragments proliferate and may, at a later date, cause mechanical bowel obstruction.[3]

(Illustration on opposite page.)

FIGURE 6.6. SPLENIC FOSSA HEMORRHAGE.

A, Plain film. G.D. had sustained multiple fractures in an automobile accident. Over the next eight days, he experienced two episodes of hypotension and falling hematocrit. This film, on the eighth day, shows a large mass in the left upper quadrant displacing the barium-filled stomach to the right. *B,* Pneumoperitoneography. The mass is adherent to the undersurface of the diaphragm. A small contracted spleen, surrounded by an estimated 1500-milliliter hematoma, was removed.
(Courtesy of Virginia Raphael, M.D., Santa Cruz Hospital, Santa Cruz, California.)

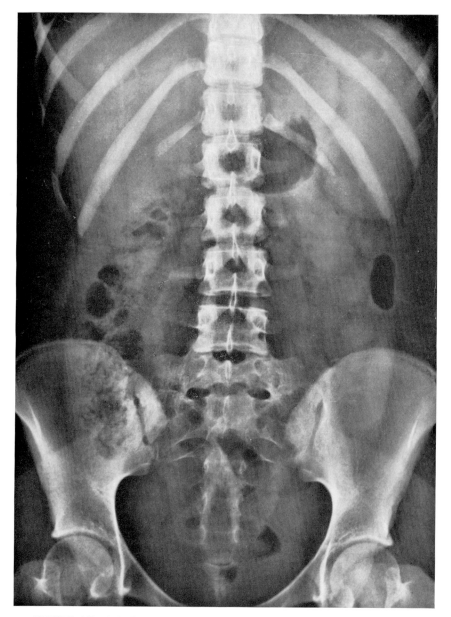

**FIGURE 6.7. SPLENIC MASS; BLOOD IN THE FLANKS AND PELVIS;
POSSIBLE BLOW-OUT OF A SUBCAPSULAR HEMATOMA.**

C.D. injured the left abdomen and five days later experienced sudden left-sided
abdominal pain. A mass in the left upper quadrant displaces the stomach and
splenic flexure. Blood is present in the flanks and in the pelvis. Kidney and psoas
outlines are intact. At operation there was a tear in the spleen suggestive of a
blow-out of a subcapsular hematoma with 500 to 700 milliliters of blood in the
peritoneum.

(Courtesy of George Hoeffler, M.D., Mills Memorial Hospital, San Mateo,
California.)

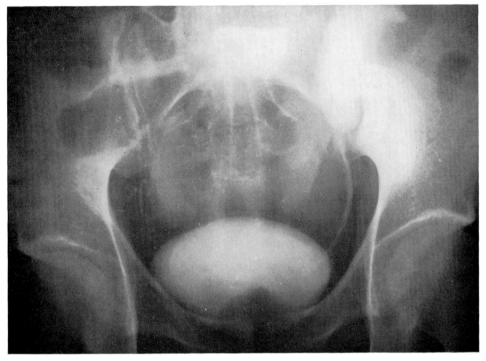

**FIGURE 6.8.   HEMOPERITONEUM FROM RUPTURED SPLEEN;
BLOOD FILLING PELVIC RECESSES.**

J.D. was unconscious after an automobile accident. He had left upper quadrant
tenderness. This radiograph shows a large accumulation of blood in the pelvic
recesses (the "dog's ears" sign). The radiographic findings were confirmed by
abdominal needle tap, and a torn spleen was removed surgically.
(Courtesy of Leon Kaseff, M.D., Franklin Hospital, San Francisco.)

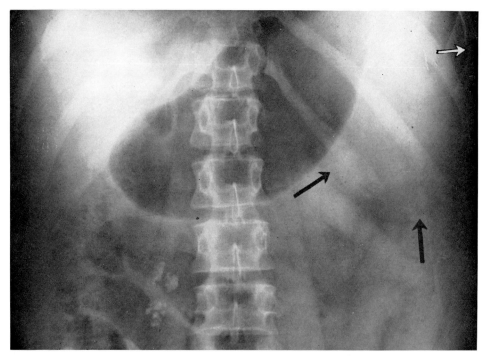

FIGURE 6.9. GASTRIC DILATION ACCOMPANYING SPLENIC RUPTURE.

J. S., a 37-year-old-man, was admitted with a bruise of the left lower anterior chest and a fracture of the left 9th rib (white arrow). In addition to marked gastric dilatation, there is a splenic mass (black arrows). Diagnosis was confirmed at operation.

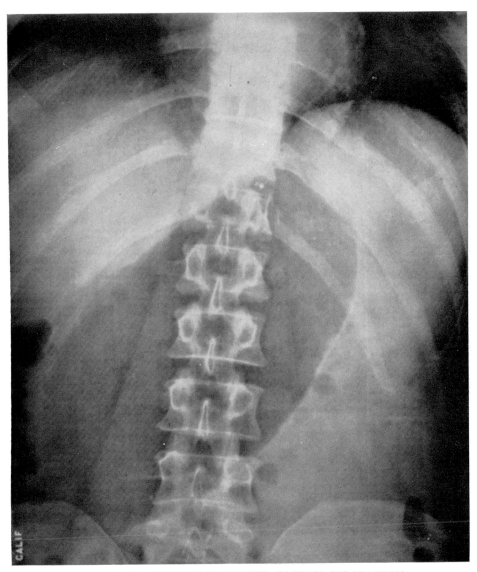

FIGURE 6.10. RUPTURED SPLEEN; GASTRIC DILATATION.

J.H. was in shock after an automobile accident. He had fractures of the left 8th, 9th and 10th ribs. Marked gastric distention with displacement of the stomach to the right side is seen. There is a splenic mass. At operation, there was a ruptured spleen and extensive intraperitoneal bleeding.

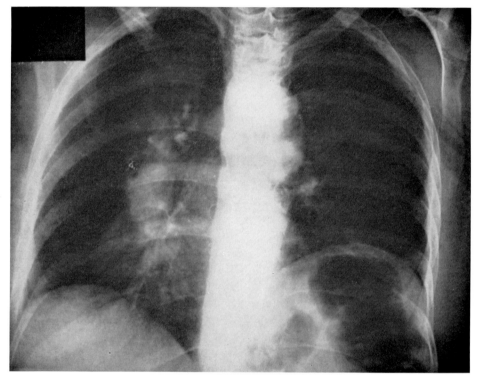

**FIGURE 6.11.   ELEVATION AND LIMITED MOBILITY OF THE LEFT LEAF OF THE
DIAPHRAGM, A SIGN OF SPLENIC LACERATION.**

E.R. sustained a fracture of the ilium with multiple contusions and lacerations.
Chest examination reveals an elevation of the left leaf of the diaphragm. A
ruptured spleen was removed.

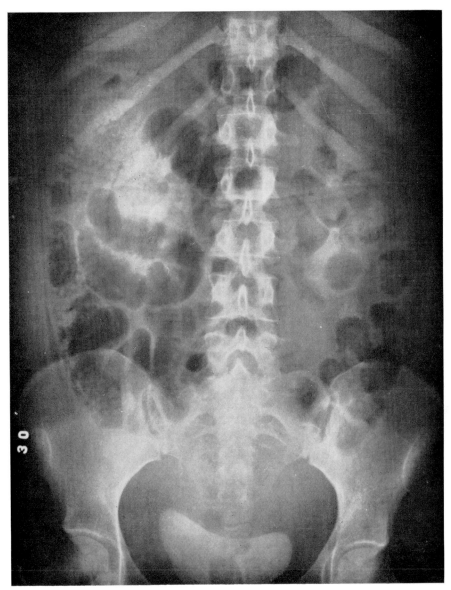

FIGURE 6.12. DELAYED RUPTURE OF THE SPLEEN (ONE WEEK).

K.C. sustained a ruptured uterus in a motorcycle accident. The uterus was repaired. At laparotomy, no other bleeding was detected. One week later, she
complained of left shoulder and flank pain. The hematocrit dropped from 30 to
26 percent in 48 hours. On this film, a mass in the left upper quadrant displaces
the stomach medially and the splenic flexure downward. A small amount of
fluid is seen in the flanks. At second laparotomy, splenic rupture was found with
free blood in the peritoneum.

REFERENCES

1. Bollinger, J. A., and Fowler, E. F.: Traumatic rupture of the spleen with special reference to delayed splenic rupture. Amer. J. Surg., *91*:561-570, 1956.
2. Cimmino, C. V.: Ruptured spleen: Some refinements in its roentgenologic diagnosis. Radiology, *82*:57, 1964.
3. Davis, C., Alexander, R. W., and De Young, H. D.: Splenosis after splenic trauma. Arch. Surg., *86*:523-533, 1963.
4. Elkin, M., and Cohen, G.: Diagnostic value of the psoas shadow. Clin. Radiol., *13*: 210-217, 1962.
5. Gershon-Cohen, J., Hermel, B., Byrne, R. M., and Bringhurst, L. S.: Rupture of the spleen. Roentgen diagnosis. Radiology, *57*:521-530, 1951.
6. Harner, M., and Chalmers, J. A.: Splenic cysts: With a report of a case. Brit. Med. J., *1*:521-523, 1946.
7. Kittredge, R. D., and Finby, N.: Infrapulmonary effusion in traumatic rupture of the spleen. Amer. J. Roentgenol., *91*:891-895, 1964.
8. Lorimer, W. S.: Occult rupture of the spleen. Arch. Surg., *89*:434-440, 1964.
9. Maughon, J. S., Geib, P. O., and Lenhardt, H. F.: Splenic trauma: An increasing problem. Surgery, *49*:477-485, 1961.
10. Pollard, J. J., and Nebesar, R. A.: Splenic rupture demonstrated by selective artery angiogram. J.A.M.A., *187*:944-945, 1964.
11. Qureshi, M. A., Hafner, C. D., and Dorchak, J. R.: Nonparasitic cysts of the spleen. Arch. Surg., *89*:570-574, 1964.
12. Sanguily, J., and Karlan, M.: Calcified pseudocyst of the spleen. Arch. Surg., *80*: 159-160, 1960.
13. Schwartz, S. S., Boley, S. J., and McKinnon, W.: The roentgen findings in traumatic rupture of the spleen in children. Amer. J. Roentgenol., *82*:505-509, 1959.
14. Shirkey, A. L., Wukash, D. C., Beal, A. C., Gordon, W. B., and DeBakey, M. E.: Surgical management of splenic injuries. Amer. J. Surg., *108*:630-635, 1964.
15. Sparkman, R. S.: Rupture of the spleen in pregnancy. Amer. J. Obst. Gynec., *76*: 587-598, 1957.
16. Steinberg, I., and Karl, R. C.: Diagnosis of rupture of the spleen by intravenous abdominal aortography. Amer. J. Roentgenol., *84*:902-906, 1960.
17. Terry, J. H.: Self, M. M., and Howard, J. M.: Injuries of the spleen. Report of 102 patients. Surgery, *40*:615-619, 1956.
18. Wang, C. C., and Robbins, L. L.: Roentgenologic diagnosis of ruptured spleen. New Engl. J. Med., *254*:445-449, 1956.
19. Wyman, A. C.: Traumatic rupture of the spleen. Amer. J. Roentgenol., *72*:51-63, 1954.
20. Zabrinski, E. J., and Harkins, H. N.: Delayed splenic rupture: A clinical syndrome following trauma. Arch. Surg., *48*:186-213, 1943.

7

LACERATION OF THE LIVER

CLINICAL OBSERVATIONS

Injury to the liver occurs in approximately 5 to 10 per cent of all patients who sustain blunt abdominal trauma. It is about half as frequent as laceration of the spleen (Table 2.1). Interestingly, the liver was the most commonly injured organ in 349 medicolegal autopsies studied by Slätis.[17] Either liver injury has a high mortality rate or minor degrees of liver injury are not diagnosed in nonfatal accidents.

In closed abdominal trauma, compression of the liver parenchyma results in jagged tears. The right lobe is injured in about four-fifths of the patients.[5, 12, 17]

The most common result of liver injury is bleeding with hemoperitoneum. This is clinically manifest by abdominal tenderness, distention and absent bowel sounds. A fall in the hematocrit is noted, and if the bleeding is continuous, shock supervenes. Only when laceration causes the bile ducts to communicate with the portal veins is melena or hematemesis found.

Liver injury may be accompanied by swelling and contusion of the soft tissues of the right upper abdomen. In the patient who is comatose or otherwise unable to give a history, injury to the soft tissues may be the only indication of the site of the blow. Serious laceration of the liver, however, can occur in the complete absence of external signs of injury. It can follow closed-chest cardiac massage (Fig. 7.7).

ASSOCIATED INJURIES

Fracture of the right lower ribs is present in almost 50 per cent of the patients.[11] Occasionally, contusion of the lung, pneumothorax and pleural bleeding are seen. Because of its anatomic proximity, contusion of the right kidney is also associated.

RADIOGRAPHIC EXAMINATION

Plain Film Examination

The inferior margin of the liver is made visible anteriorly by adjacent mesenteric fat and posteriorly, in part, by the perirenal fat. In injury to the liver, the outline of the inferior margin of the liver is lost; severe trauma is unlikely if the sharp margin of the undersurface of the liver is seen. Loss of liver outline can be due to technical factors, and its absence is not of diagnostic significance.

Opacification of Stomach and Bowel

A subcapsular hematoma on the undersurface of the liver may displace the stomach or the transverse colon. If these structures are not identifiable, barium or water-soluble iodide solution is administered.

Arteriography

Because bleeding is a prominent feature of liver injury, arteriography is an excellent method of demonstrating subcapsular or parenchymal extravasation. It is accomplished by catheterization of the celiac axis.

Pneumoperitoneography

The outline of the liver is well shown by pneumoperitoneum. Films are taken in the prone, supine and left lateral decubitus projections.

Radioactive Isotope Scanning

In the presence of hematobilia, a central laceration can be identified by radioactive isotope scanning. Given intravenously, colloidal radioactive gold accumulates in the reticuloendothelial system of the liver, or I^{131}-tagged rose bengal is excreted by the polygonal cells. A focus of low activity indicates cellular necrosis.

Fluoroscopy of Diaphragmatic Movement

Since injury to the liver may be accompanied by contusion of the right leaf of the diaphragm or the accumulation of fluid between the dome of the liver and the diaphragm, the right leaf is studied by fluoroscopy or by serial chest films. When elevation of the right leaf is found, the differential diagnosis is made between rupture, subdiaphragmatic hematoma and diaphragmatic splinting due to muscle spasm. With rupture of the diaphragm, the motion is paradoxical and the liver edge is high in position. With subdiaphragmatic hematoma, the motion of the diaphragm is limited and the liver edge is either in its normal position or slightly lower than normal. Splinting of the diaphragm due to contusion causes limitation of motion with no change in the position of the liver edge.

Operative Cholangiography

To outline the biliary tree at time of operation, 15 to 20 milliliters of 25 per cent diatrizoate sodium are injected by needle puncture or polyethylene catheter into the common duct. This examination will reveal central laceration and will define the extent of the injury to the hepatic ducts.

TYPES OF LIVER INJURY

Radiographically, four major types of bleeding are encountered: (1) subcapsular hematoma, (2) localized subdiaphragmatic hematoma, (3) central laceration with hematobilia and (4) intraperitoneal bleeding.

Subcapsular Hematoma

Subcapsular hematoma occurs when the liver is torn beneath the intact capsule. It is more common in children. When the hematoma presents anteriorly, a mass in the right upper quadrant is palpable.

Radiographically, subcapsular hematoma on the undersurface of the liver appears as a bulge of the liver indenting the transverse colon (Fig. 7.1). On arteriography, the peripheral branches of the hepatic artery are spread out by the enlarging hematoma (Fig. 7.2). Clinical or radiologic findings of subcapsular hematoma are an indication for surgical drainage.[1]

Localized Hematoma

A small tear of the capsule of the liver with limited bleeding causes the formation of localized hematoma. This was seen in one patient who had a hematoma between the diaphragm and the dome of the liver (Fig. 7.3). The dome of the diaphragm was elevated, but the inferior edge of

(Text continued on page 99)

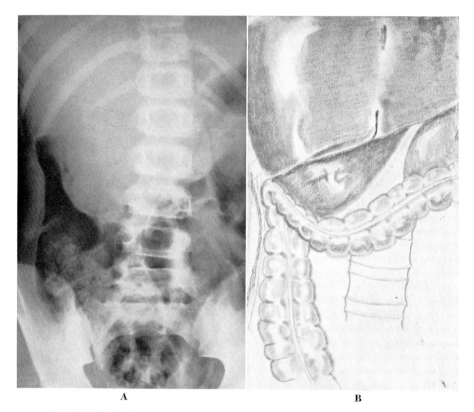

A   B

**FIGURE 7.1. SUBCAPSULAR HEMATOMA OF LIVER DISPLACING
TRANSVERSE COLON.**

A, Plain film. After a fall, this child (J.P.) had severe pain in the right upper
quadrant. A mass continuous with the liver compresses and displaces the hepatic
flexure of the colon downward and laterally. *B,* Diagram. At operation, a large
subcapsular hematoma containing 200 to 400 milliliters of dark blood was opened
and aspirated.

(Illustration on opposite page.)

**FIGURE 7.2. SUBCAPSULAR HEMATOMA OF LIVER DEMONSTRATED BY
CELIAC ARTERIOGRAPHY.**

A, Arterial phase. B.U. injured the right upper abdomen. A celiac arteriogram
was obtained by retrograde femoral catheterization. The arterial phase shows
an avascular area in the right lobe of the liver with displacement of the hepatic
artery and its branches. *B,* Capillary phase. The hematoma is less dense
than the surrounding liver parenchyma. There are no abnormal vessels to suggest a tumor. At operation, a large subcapsular hematoma was evacuated.
(Courtesy of Tord Olin, M.D., Lund, Sweden.)

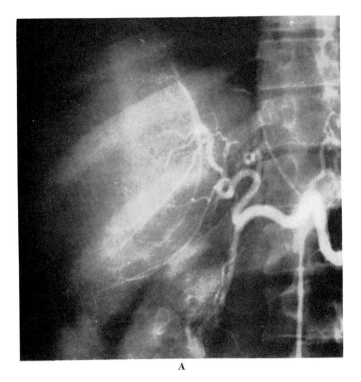

A

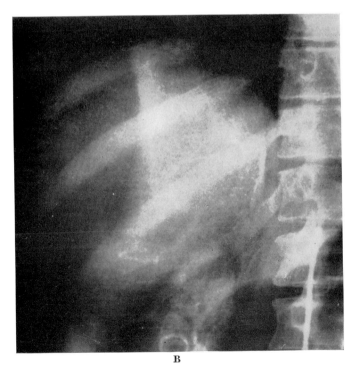

B

Figure 7.2. *See legend on opposite page.*

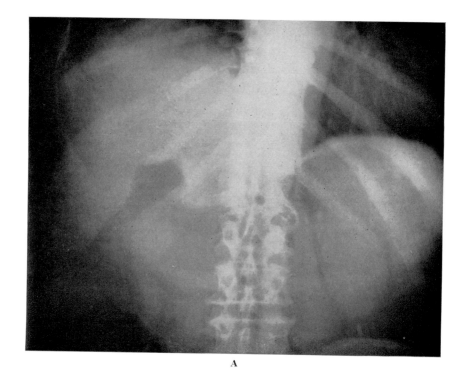

A

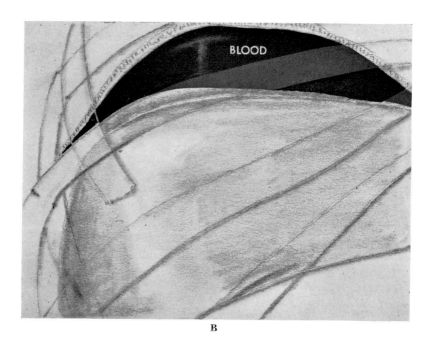

B

Figure 7.3. *See legend on opposite page*

the liver was in its normal position, differentiating it from right diaphragmatic tear in which the liver is elevated.

Central Laceration with Hematobilia

Traumatic hemobilia was the name given to this type of injury by
Sandblom[14] in 1948. It is the least common type of injury. Central
laceration produces a communication between the portal system and the
biliary tree. Subsequent bleeding into the intestinal tract may be intermittent and is manifest by hematemesis, melena and bilary colic. Sparkman[19] found a close time relationship between the pain and bleeding.
Usually, the onset of pain was accompanied or followed by melena. Twenty-
two of 42 reported cases have been due to nonpenetrating injury.[18] Three
characteristics of traumatic hematobilia are said to make the diagnosis
difficult: (1) delay of several weeks after trauma in the appearance of
bleeding, (2) periodicity of the bleeding episodes and (3) confusion of the
clinical picture by previous operation.

Schatzki[15] has described a diagnostic triad of abdominal pain suggestive
of biliary colic, gastrointestinal bleeding and a history of trauma. He
recommends study of the patient by (1) scintillation survey of the liver,
(2) retrograde catheterization of the aorta with opacification of the hepatic
artery, (3) operative hepatic arteriogram and (4) operative cholangiography.
In the case reported by Schatzki, the operative cholangiogram showed a
hepatic duct to terminate in a large irregular cavity (Fig. 7.4).

By means of radioactive isotope scanning Ruskin and Saenger[13] have
detected a central laceration causing hemobilia. Scanograms show a filling
defect within the liver substance after a tracer dose of I^{131}-labeled rose
bengal (Fig. 7.5).

Free Intraperitoneal Bleeding

This is the most common sequel to liver injury. Blood accumulates
in the flank between the peritoneal fat line and the ascending and descending segments of the colon (Figs. 7.6 and 7.7). In some cases this is more

(*Text continued on page 104*)

(Illustration on opposite page.)

**FIGURE 7.3. LOCALIZED SUBDIAPHRAGMATIC HEMATOMA;
ELEVATED RIGHT LEAF OF DIAPHRAGM.**

A, Plain film. J.P. had been struck by an auto. Radiographic examination shows
fractures of the right 8th and 9th ribs. The right leaf of the diaphragm is elevated. *B*, Diagram. He died shortly after admission, and at autopsy there was
a collection of blood interposed between the dome of the liver and the diaphragm.
(From McCort, J. J.: Rupture or laceration of the liver by nonpenetrating
trauma. Radiology, *78*:49-57, 1962.)

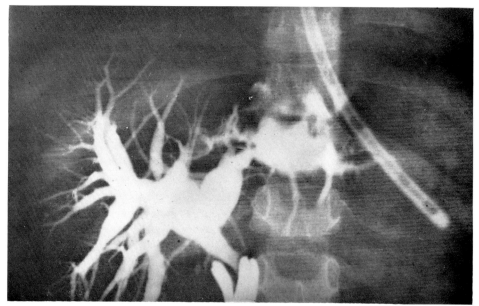

**FIGURE 7.4. CENTRAL LACERATION OF LIVER WITH HEMOBILIA;
OPERATIVE CHOLANGIOGRAM.**

Fourteen days after injury, this child developed severe abdominal pain, accompanied by hepatomegaly and jaundice. Eighteen and 21 days following injury, massive gastrointestinal hemorrhages occurred. An exploratory laparotomy revealed enlargement of the left lobe of the liver. The left hepatic artery was ligated. The hematemesis and melena continued. Three months later, at the laparotomy, this operative cholangiogram shows the left hepatic duct to communicate with a necrotic area.
(From Schatzki, S. C.: Hemobilia. Radiology, *77*:717-721, 1961.)

(Illustration on opposite page.)

FIGURE 7.5. CENTRAL LACERATION OF LIVER WITH HEMATOBILIA.

A, Liver scan. K.B. Seven days after contusion of the abdomen, he complained of abdominal pain and vomited blood. At laparotomy, a laceration of the right lobe of the liver was sutured. He improved and was discharged. Thirty days later he again vomited bright red blood. On the liver scan, a filling defect in the right lobe of the liver is seen. Intermittent bouts of colicky pain, jaundice and melena continued. The patient died following a right hepatic lobectomy. *B,* Injected specimen. The radiograph of the injected autopsy specimen shows an area of necrosis corresponding to the defect demonstrated on the scan.
(From Ruskin, R., and Saenger, E. L.: Liver scanning in the diagnosis of hematobilia. Radiology, *81*:980-982, 1963.)

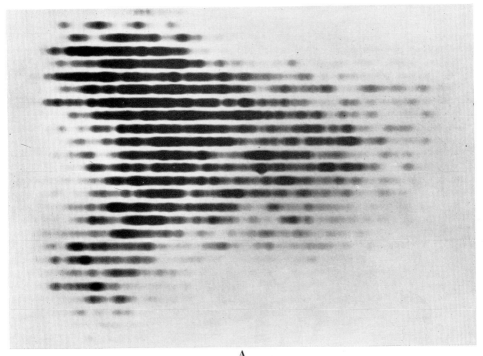

A

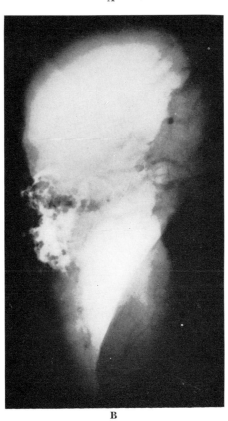

B

Figure 7.5. *See legend on opposite page.*

101

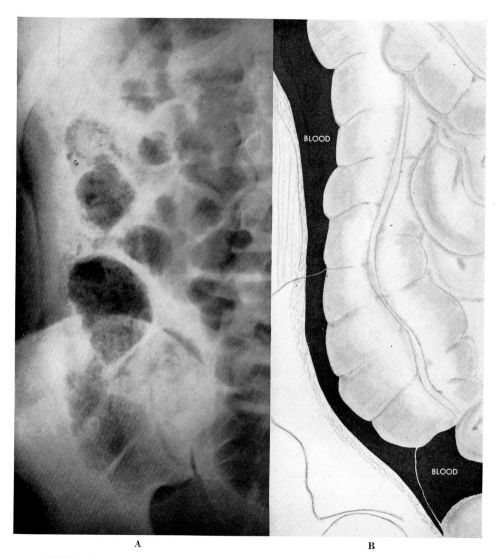

A   B

**FIGURE 7.6. LIVER LACERATION WITH INTRAPERITONEAL BLEEDING;
BLOOD IN FLANK.**

A, Anteroposterior. E.G. After an automobile accident he had severe right-sided
abdominal pain. Intraperitoneal blood is present on the right side between the
fat line and the ascending colon.   *B,* Diagram. At operation there was a laceration of the right lobe of the liver with approximately 700 milliliters of free blood
throughout the abdomen.

(From McCort, J. J.: Rupture or laceration of the liver by nonpenetrating
trauma. Radiology, *78:*49-57, 1962.)

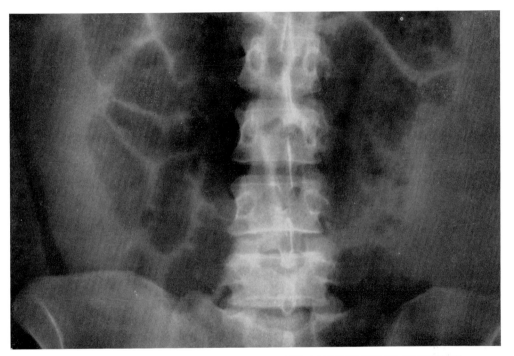

**FIGURE 7.7. LIVER LACERATION WITH INTRAPERITONEAL BLEEDING;
SEQUEL TO EXTERNAL CARDIAC MASSAGE.**

L.V.B. Two days after vaginal hysterectomy, the patient had cardiac arrest. External cardiac massage was begun immediately and there was a return of cardiac
contractions, blood pressure and level of consciousness. Subsequently, blood
pressure and hematocrit declined and the patient compained of epigastric and
right shoulder pain. A large amount of blood is present in both flanks and the
loops of small bowel are clustered in the midline. The intraperitoneal bleeding
was due to a stellate laceration of the liver.

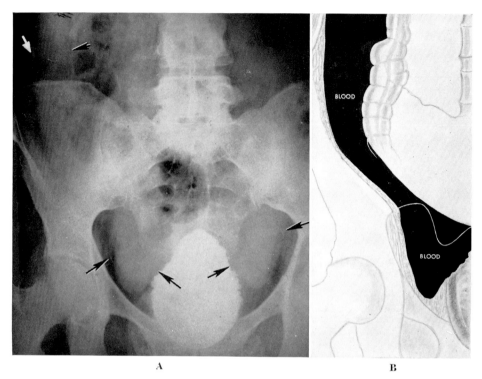

A   B

FIGURE 7.8. LIVER LACERATION WITH INTRAPERITONEAL BLEEDING.

A, Anteroposterior. N.C. This patient had fractures of the right 6th, 7th and 8th ribs in the midaxillary line. A large amount of blood is seen in the right side of the abdomen between the fat line and ascending colon (upper arrows) and in the pelvis on both sides of the bladder (lower arrows) ("dog's ears" sign). *B,* Diagram. Bleeding was due to a 6-inch laceration of the right lobe of the liver. There were about 2000 milliliters of blood in the peritoneal cavity.
(From McCort, J. J.: Rupture or laceration of the liver by nonpenetrating trauma. Radiology, *78:*49-57, 1962.)

noticeable on the right side. Blood is also seen in the peritoneal recesses of the pelvis (Figs. 7.8 and 7.9).

McClelland, Shires and Poulos[10] report a high diagnostic accuracy with abdominal paracentesis for the diagnosis of intra-abdominal bleeding and liver injury. In 22 of 31 blunt injury patients who had peritoneal tap, there was only one failure to reveal nonclotting blood.

Shaftan, Gliedman and Cappelletti[16] found the mortality of liver injuries proportional to the amount of hemoperitoneum. With no bleeding

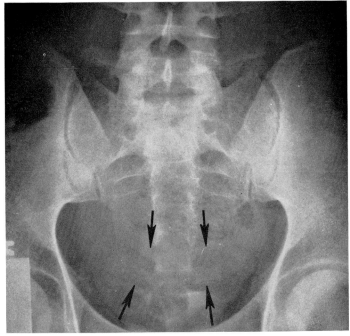

A

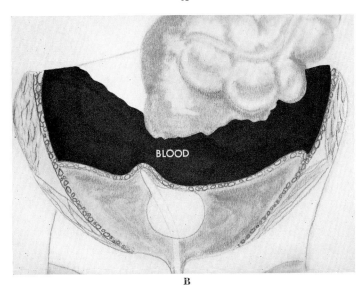

B

FIGURE 7.9. LIVER LACERATION WITH INTRAPERITONEAL BLEEDING.

A, Anteroposterior. J.L. had fractures of the right 8th, 9th and 10th ribs laterally, and there was a small amount of blood in the pleural space. Blood was also seen in the flanks between the colon and the fat line. On this film, a Foley catheter is present in the bladder. *B,* Diagram. Blood is present in the pelvic recesses and is interposed between the rectosigmoid colon and the bladder (arrows).
(From McCort, J. J.: Rupture or laceration of the liver by nonpenetrating trauma. Radiology, *78:*49-57, 1962.)

it was zero, and with increasing amounts of blood, it rose steeply. With more than 3000 milliliters of blood in the peritoneum, the mortality was 100 per cent.

DELAYED RUPTURE OF THE LIVER

This phenomenon is less frequent than delayed rupture of diaphragm or spleen. Follow-up films, when compared with those taken initially, show an accumulation of blood in the flanks and pelvis (Fig. 7.10).

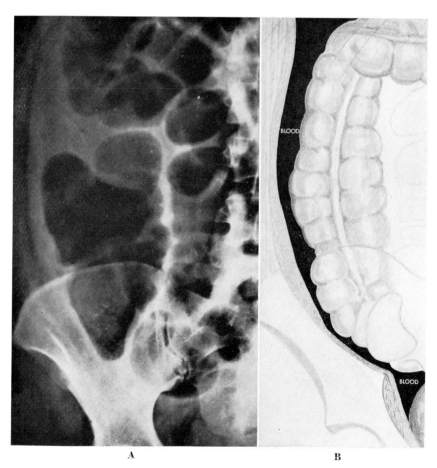

A   B

FIGURE 7.10. DELAYED RUPTURE OF THE LIVER (7 DAYS AFTER INJURY).

A, Anteroposterior. After an automobile accident, M.D. had multiple fractures and lacerations. On admission, there were no abnormal physical and radiographic findings in the abdomen. Six days later, she developed increasing abdominal distention with absent peristalsis. Her hemoglobin dropped to 8.2 grams. This abdominal film, on the 7th day, shows blood in the flank and pelvis. *B,* Diagram. At operation, the peritoneal cavity contained one liter of blood from a liver laceration.

COMPLICATIONS OF LIVER LACERATION

Liver Necrosis

Post-traumatic necrosis of the liver has been found in two cases at the Santa Clara County Hospital. Even though the laceration is repaired and bleeding stopped, a traumatized segment of the liver may be sufficiently devitalized to undergo necrosis. Superimposed infection will result in abscess formation. Radiographically, a collection of small bubbles outlines the necrotic liver segment (Fig. 7.11).

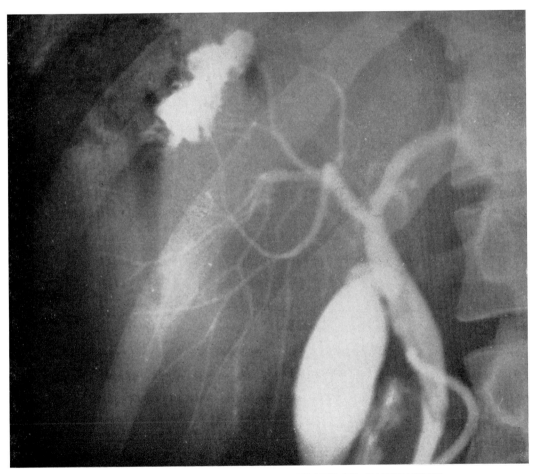

FIGURE 7.11. LIVER ABSCESS SECONDARY TO LACERATION; T-TUBE CHOLANGIOGRAPHY.

F.L. struck his abdomen against the steering wheel. At operation, a liver laceration was found and repaired. Two weeks later, the laceration of the liver became infected. T-tube drainage was performed. On T-tube cholangiography, the injected opaque medium extravasates into a hepatic abscess. The abscess cleared on tube drainage and antibiotics.
(Courtesy of George Jacobson, M.D., Los Angeles County Hospital, Los Angeles, California.)

Subdiaphragmatic or Subhepatic Abscess

Patients who have rupture of the liver that seals spontaneously may later develop subphrenic or subhepatic abscess (Figs. 7.12 and 7.13). Cameron and Sykes[2] report three cases of subphrenic abscess following trauma and without perforation of the gastrointestinal tract. Two occurrences followed rupture of the liver and one a ruptured spleen. All three patients had intra-abdominal hemorrhage.

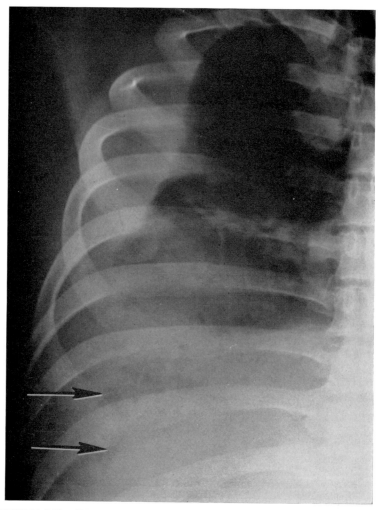

FIGURE 7.12. SUBDIAPHRAGMATIC ABSCESS AND LIVER NECROSIS FOLLOWING LACERATION.

T.K. struck his abdomen against the steering wheel and was found to have blood in the peritoneal cavity. A large "Y"-shaped laceration of the dome of the liver was repaired. On the 5th postoperative day, a right pleural effusion and paralytic ileus developed. A collection of small bubbles of gas indicates necrosis with infection (arrows). On surgical exploration, an area of necrosis in the right lobe was drained.

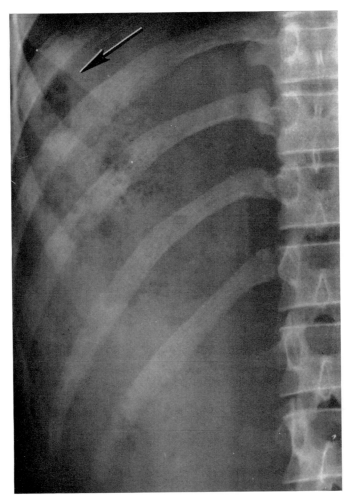

FIGURE 7.13. SUBHEPATIC ABSCESS FROM RUPTURE OF THE LIVER.

R.B., after an automobile accident, he was found to have a ruptured liver with subhepatic collection of blood. The liver laceration was repaired and the blood drained. Twelve days later, he complained of a colicky pain. A mottling due to multiple small bubbles of gas mixed with fluid is seen in the subhepatic area (arrow). The wound was reopened. Liquid and clotted blood mixed with bile was drained from beneath the liver.

Post-traumatic Liver Cyst

This is a rare occurrence. A patient is reported by Kerekes and Ewing[6] in whom the entire right lobe of the liver was replaced by a fibrous walled cyst.

LACERATION OF THE EXTRAHEPATIC BILE DUCTS

Patients with this unusual injury are in a profound state of shock.[8] Spontaneous recovery may occur, followed after an interval of several days by jaundice, dark urine and light stool. Mason, Sidbury and Guiang[9] point out that jaundice with an acholic stool is a constant finding in rupture of the bile duct, whereas it is rare in rupture of the liver. The usual site of a rupture of the common duct is at the superior border of the pancreas.[3, 7] With the escape of bile into the peritoneum, there are clinical and radiographic signs of peritonitis.

LACERATION OF THE GALLBLADDER

This is an uncommon injury as a result of blunt trauma. Hall et al.[4] observed 25 patients with injury to the gallbladder in a 15-year period. Only two of the injuries were due to blunt trauma. Bile peritonitis is the usual result.

REFERENCES

1. Brittain, R. S.: Liver trauma. Surg. Clin. North America, *43*:433-443, 1963.
2. Cameron, D. A., and Sykes, E. M.: Subphrenic abscess in trauma. Amer. J. Surg., *83:* 412-426, 1952.
3. Fletcher, W. S., Mahnke, D. E., and Dunphy, J. E.: Complete division of the common bile duct due to blunt trauma. J. Trauma, *1*:87-95, 1961.
4. Hall, E. R., Howard, J. M., Jordan, G. L., and Mikesky, W. E.: Traumatic injuries of the gallbladder. A.M.A. Arch. Surg., *72*:520-524, 1956.
5. Hellström, G.: Closed injury of the liver. Acta Chir. Scand., *122*:490-501, 1961.
6. Kerekes, E. S., and Ewing, J.: Traumatic liver cyst. Radiology, *55*:861-864, 1950.
7. Lee, J. G., and Wherry, D. C.: Traumatic rupture of the extra-hepatic biliary ducts from external trauma. J. Trauma, *1*:105-114, 1961.
8. Lewis, K. M.: Traumatic rupture of the bile ducts. Ann. Surg., *108*:237-242, 1938.
9. Mason, L. B., Sidbury, J. B., and Guiang, S.: Rupture of the extrahepatic bile ducts from non-penetrating trauma. Ann. Surg., *140*:234-241, 1954.
10. McClelland, R., Shires, T., and Poulos, E.: Hepatic resection for massive trauma. J. Trauma, *4*:282-291, 1964.
11. McCort, J. J.: Rupture or laceration of the liver by non-penetrating trauma. Radiology, *77*:717-721, 1961.
12. Mikesky, W. E., Howard, J. M., and DeBakey, M. E.: Injuries of the liver in 300 consecutive patients. Int. Abstr. Surg., *103*:323-337, 1956.
13. Ruskin, R., and Saenger, E. L.: Liver scanning in the diagnosis of hematobilia. Radiology, *81*:980-982, 1963.

14. Sandblom, P.: Hemorrhage into the biliary tract following trauma. Traumatic hemobilia. Surgery, *24*:571-586, 1948.
15. Schatzki, S. C.: Hemobilia. Radiology, *77*:717-721, 1961.
16. Shaftan, G. W., Gliedman, M. L., and Cappelletti, R. R.: Injuries of the liver. A review of 111 cases. J. Trauma, *3*:61-72, 1963.
17. Slätis, P.: Injuries in fatal traffic accidents. An analysis of 349 medicolegal autopsies. Acta Chir. Scand., Suppl. 297, Stockholm, 1962.
18. Souliotis, P. T., Pettigrew, A. H., and Chamberlain, J. W.: Traumatic hemobilia. N. Engl. J. Med., *268*:565-568, 1963.
19. Sparkman, R. S.: Massive hemobilia following traumatic rupture of liver. Ann. Surg., *138*:899-910, 1953.

8

LACERATION OF THE MESENTERY

CLINICAL OBSERVATIONS

Laceration of the mesentery is usually seen in association with multiple visceral injuries, but occasionally it occurs alone. It varies in severity from minor contusion to an extensive through-and-through tear. With slight injury, the hematoma formed in the mesentery is self-limited. The patient has mild symptoms and quickly recovers.

With larger mesenteric tears, the arteries and veins supplying the bowel are disrupted. Usually the patient complains of persistent abdominal pain. Clinical evidence of bleeding into the peritoneal cavity includes abdominal distention, absence of bowel sounds, incipient shock and a falling hematocrit.

When a segment of the bowel loses its blood supply and the collateral circulation is inadequate, the bowel becomes gangrenous. This situation is signaled by shock, abdominal distention and bloody diarrhea. If perforation of the gangrenous segment takes place, the signs of a diffuse septic peritonitis are superimposed.

Spontaneous healing can take place if a limited segment of the bowel has been devascularized. At a later date, contracture of the fibrous tissue replacing the necrotic bowel may cause mechanical obstruction.

112

INTRAPERITONEAL BLEEDING

Free intraperitoneal bleeding follows tearing of the serosa and mesenteric vessels. It is recognized by the presence of blood in the flanks and pelvis, by the flotation of the small bowel loops and by the separation of the bowel loops (Figs. 8.1 and 8.2). *The site of the bleeding cannot be*

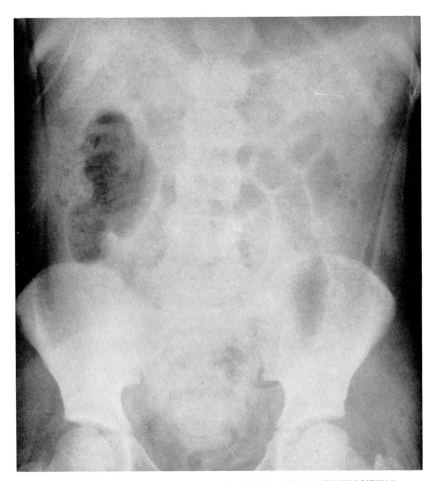

FIGURE 8.1. MESENTERIC LACERATION; HEMOPERITONEUM.

S.Z., after an automobile accident, had absence of bowel sounds and increasing abdominal tenderness. This film, at 24 hours, shows blood in the right flank between the ascending colon and the properitoneal fat. None is seen on the left. At laparotomy, there was between 400 and 500 milliliters of blood in the peritoneal cavity from a transverse tear in the small bowel mesentery. The ileum adjacent to the lacerated mesentery was ischemic.

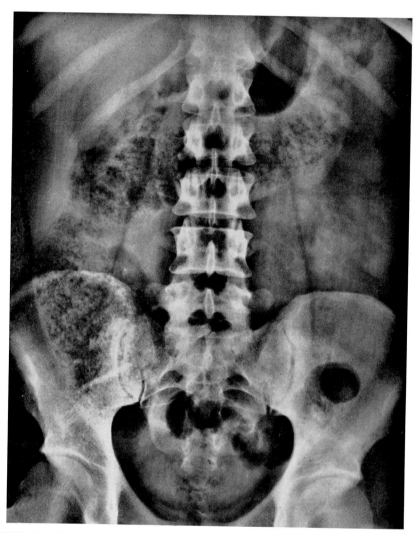

FIGURE 8.2. LACERATION OF THE JEJUNAL MESENTERY; HEMOPERITONEUM.

J.G. had been thrown from a car and was unconscious when found. Blood is seen in the pelvic recesses and left flank. At operation, 2000 milliliters of blood in the peritoneal cavity was found to have come from two lacerated and actively bleeding jejunal arteries. Despite the large amount of blood in the peritoneal cavity of this patient, the kidney and psoas muscles are sharply outlined. Intraperitoneal hemorrhage does not obscure the retroperitoneal structures.

determined on the basis of the plain radiograph. Rupture of the mesenteric vessels could conceivably be detected by arteriography of the superior and inferior mesenteric arteries; no such studies have been reported.

AVASCULAR NECROSIS OF THE BOWEL WITH PERFORATION

With wide and severe tears of the mesentery, the viability of the bowel is compromised by the loss of its blood supply. Changes in the bowel wall vary from severe swelling to actual necrosis and gangrene. The bowel wall becomes thickened by edema and inflammatory exudation. Denudation of the mucosal surface results in large irregular ulcers.[3] The speed of progression of these changes is proportional to the severity of the injury and the duration of the avascular period. Radiographically, the thick wall of a necrotic segment may be visible if the segment is distended with gas (Fig. 8.3). The mucosal surface is irregular and gas may be seen in the wall of the bowel. Perforation of the necrotic segment causes fulminating peritonitis.[2, 5] Because the bowel has an extensive collateral blood supply, avascular necrosis is an uncommon finding in mesenteric trauma.

McCune et al.[4] reported four cases of mesenteric venous thrombosis following blunt abdominal trauma and noted these characteristics: (1) The thrombus continues to extend even after resection of an infarcted segment of bowel, and unless all of the mesenteric thrombus has been removed, an extension of the gangrenous process may result. (2) Rate of propagation of the thrombus is variable; infarction may occur up to five weeks after injury. (3) Separate thrombi in various parts of the venous mesentery may extend at different rates.

POST-TRAUMATIC STENOSIS OF THE BOWEL

When only a small segment of the bowel is devascularized, the course may be relatively benign. The small infarcted segment undergoes cicatrization (Fig. 8.4). Radiographically, there is an annular narrowing of the involved segment[6, 8] with mucosal ulceration. Within a period of weeks or months, signs and symptoms of intestinal obstruction appear. The lesions resemble those which result from mesenteric thrombosis or embolism.[1, 7]

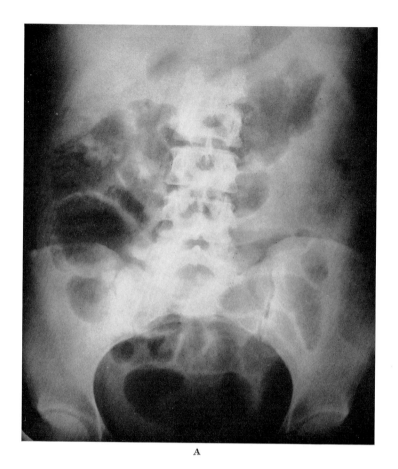

A

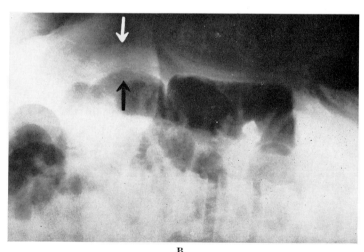

B

Figure 8.3. *See legend on opposite page.*

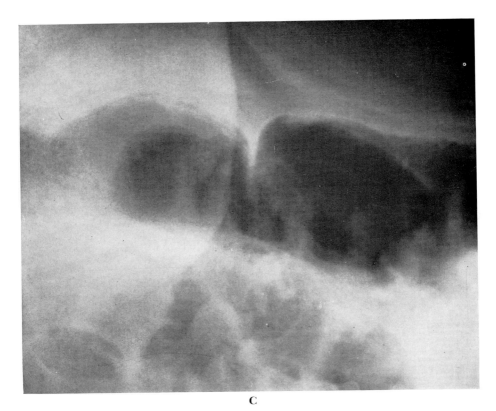

C

FIGURE 8.3. AVULSION OF MESENTERIC VESSELS WITH INFARCTION OF THE ASCENDING COLON.

A, Supine film. J.P. jumped from a 40-foot bridge and sustained multiple contusions and abrasions. The supine film of the abdomen shows blood in the flanks and pelvis. *B,* Left lateral decubitus film. In the lateral decubitus projection, the wall of the cecum is outlined by the intracolic gas and is nodular and thickened (arrows). *C,* Cecal wall. At operation, the abdomen contained 1000 milliliters of bloody fluid. The right colon was gangrenous.

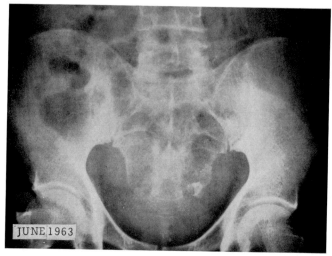

JUNE 1963

A

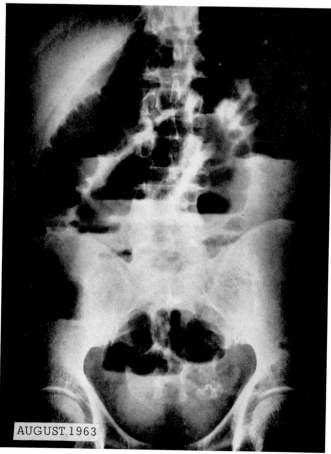

AUGUST 1963

B

FIGURE 8.4. CICATRIZATION OF THE SMALL BOWEL DUE TO MESENTERIC VASCULAR INJURY; SUBSEQUENT INTESTINAL OBSTRUCTION.

A, Initial. Plain film. M.R. had been kicked in the abdomen during a fight. The initial film shows blood in the pelvis. After several blood transfusions his con-

(Continued on next page)

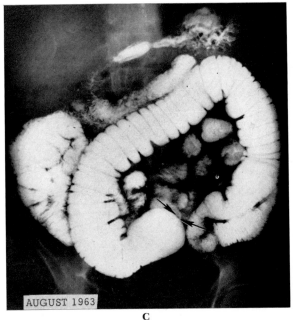

AUGUST 1963

C

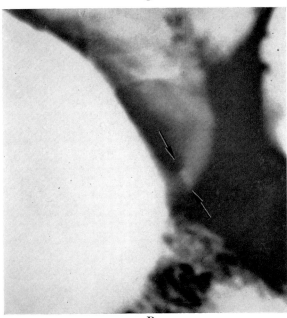

D

Figure 8.4. *Continued.*

dition stabilized. No surgical treatment was carried out. *B,* Plain film, 2 months later, at which time he was re-admitted with abdominal distention and vomiting. There are dilated loops of small bowel containing gas and fluid, indicating small bowel obstruction. *C,* Barium study of small bowel. After nasogastric tube aspiration for 3 days, he was given barium by mouth. An abrupt constriction of the lumen of the bowel in the midjejunum is seen (arrows) with a small central ulceration. *D,* Spot film of stenotic area. On exploration, a 2-inch length of distal jejunum was involved in a circumferential scar. Several hematomas were found in the mesentery. (The patient had no clinical evidence of heart disease and had not been taking enteric-coated medication.)

119

REFERENCES

1. Hawkins, C. F.: Jejunal stenosis following mesenteric artery occlusion. Lancet, *273:* 121-122, 1957.
2. Hinckley, H. M., and Albertson, H. A.: Avulsion of the mesentery with gangrene of a segment of small bowel (ileum) following nonpenetrating trauma of abdomen. Ann. Surg., *140:*257-259, 1954.
3. Hughes, L. E., and Smaill, P. B.: Long-delayed complications of closed abdominal trauma. Brit. Med. J., *1:*776-777, 1962.
4. McCune, W. S., Keshishian, J. M., and Blades, B. B.: Mesenteric thrombosis following blunt abdominal trauma. Ann. Surg., *135:*606-614, 1952.
5. Penn, I., and Mendels, J.: Gangrene of the caecum following closed abdominal injury. Brit. J. Surg., *50:*112-113, 1962.
6. Peyini, G.: Considerazione su di un caso di stenosi del tenue post traumatica. Policlinico (sez. chir.), *39:*847-851, 1952.
7. Rosenman, L. D., and Gropper, A. W.: Small intestine stenosis caused by infarction: An unusual sequel of mesenteric artery embolism. Ann. Surg., *141:*254-262, 1955.
8. Wolf, B. S., and Marshak, R. H.: Segmental infarction of the small bowel. Radiology, *69:*701-707, 1956.

9

LACERATION OF THE INTESTINAL TRACT

CLINICAL OBSERVATIONS

When a sudden blow compresses the anterior abdominal wall, the intestine is squeezed against the rigid vertebrae. Experimental studies by Williams and Sargent[31] show that portions of the bowel more or less fixed in relation to the spine, such as the duodenojejunal junction, proximal jejunum, terminal ileum and the transverse and sigmoid colon, are more likely to sustain injury.

Three types of intestinal injury follow blunt trauma: (1) intramural hemorrhage with or without obstruction, (2) intraperitoneal perforation or (3) retroperitoneal perforation.

Intramural hemorrhage is most common in the upper small bowel. Following the traumatic episode, the hematoma in the bowel wall slowly enlarges, compromising the lumen of the bowel. Within a few hours to several days, symptoms of high intestinal obstruction appear.[4, 13, 18, 26, 30] Because only a small amount of intestinal bleeding will occlude the lumen, blood loss is minimal and the hematocrit remains stable.[25] A hematoma around the ampulla of Vater can cause common duct obstruction and jaundice.[8]

With intraperitoneal perforation, air and food particles in various stages of digestion are emptied into the peritoneal space and signs of peritonitis develop rapidly. The abdomen is distended and peristalsis is absent. There is diffuse tenderness and muscle guarding.

121

With a retroperitoneal perforation, the inflammatory process tends to be localized and abscess frequently develops.

ASSOCIATED INJURIES

In patients seen at the Santa Clara County Hospital, there was no definite pattern of associated injuries. In 18 patients with laceration of the jejunum and ileum, 3 had a fracture of the pelvis, and 2 had an associated tear of the omentum and mesentery. Three patients with rupture of the splenic flexure had fractures of the left lower ribs.

Kerry and Glas[17] found duodenal rupture frequently associated with pancreatic contusion. In the cases they reviewed, the mortality of perforated duodenum was 54 per cent.

Visceral rupture, particularly of the stomach and small intestine, found in infants and small children is at times due to abuse by parents or other adults (Fig. 9.10). The children are often unkempt and malnourished and show multiple contusions and bruises.[20] A roentgenologic survey of the skeleton and skull discloses old and new fractures, further evidence of repeated trauma. To avoid further injury, an abused and battered child must either be protected or removed from the hazardous environment.

RADIOGRAPHIC EXAMINATION

Plain Film Examination

Plain film examination, particularly the decubitus projection, is helpful in intraperitoneal perforation. It will show the presence of air, fluid or food particles outside the intestinal tract. If only the supine film is available, the presence of the dome sign, visualization of the falciform ligament or of the outer wall of the bowel, indicates intraperitoneal air. Air outside the intestinal tract is sufficient indication for immediate operation.

Gastrointestinal Examination

If the patient has persistent vomiting following abdominal trauma or if injury to the upper intestinal tract is suspected and no free air is found, the stomach and small bowel are studied with barium sulfate solution or a water-soluble medium.

Colon Examination

The colon is examined with a 25 per cent solution of diatrizoate sodium if the patient is passing blood by rectum and there is no free air in the peritoneal cavity.

LACERATION OF THE STOMACH

Rupture of the stomach occurs rarely and was seen in only three patients, all children. Because the stomach has a thick muscular wall, is freely movable and is not fixed in relation to the spine, it is resistant to compressive injuries.[1] Gastric distention following a heavy meal may make the stomach more susceptible to rupture.

With gastric rupture, a large amount of gas and fluid fills the peritoneal cavity (Fig. 9.1).

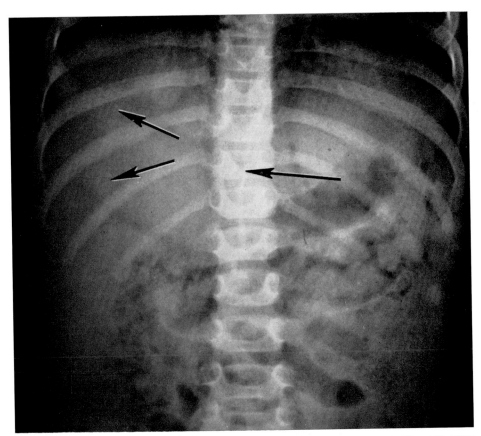

FIGURE 9.1. RUPTURE OF THE STOMACH CAUSING AIR AND FLUID IN THE PERITONEAL CAVITY; THE "DOME SIGN" AND THE "FALCIFORM LIGAMENT SIGN."

K.W., a 4-year-old girl, was run over by a truck. This radiograph shows an interface between air and fluid in the peritoneal cavity (short arrows), the "dome sign." Air is seen on both sides of the falciform ligament (long arrow). The air and fluid in the peritoneum came from a 4-inch tear in the stomach.

LACERATION OF THE DUODENUM

Because the duodenum is partially retroperitoneal, it is fixed in relation to the spine and is more vulnerable to blunt injury. In order of frequency, duodenal injury can be manifest by: (1) intramural hematoma, (2) retroperitoneal perforation or (3) intraperitoneal perforation.

Intramural Hematoma of the Duodenum

The appearance of a duodenal hematoma varies with its size and location. Duodenal hematoma may present as: (1) a filling defect in the wall of the bowel, (2) a flattening and widening of the mucosal folds, (3) a concentric narrowing with partial or complete obstruction to the canal.

FILLING DEFECT IN WALL OF BOWEL. A small localized hematoma in one side of the wall projects into the lumen and resembles a small bowel tumor (Fig. 9.2). It has been likened to a thumb print.

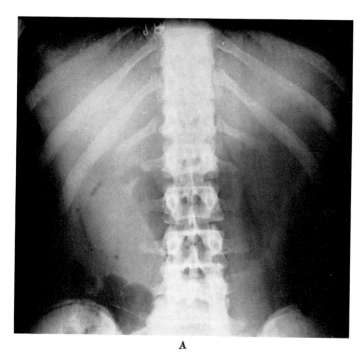

A

FIGURE 9.2.   INTRAMURAL HEMATOMA OF THE DUODENUM; FILLING DEFECT IN BOWEL WALL.

A, Preliminary film. M.J., a 15-year-old girl, was kicked in the mid-abdomen by a horse. Shortly thereafter, she became nauseated and suffered severe pain. This film shows an epigastric mass outlined by gas in the duodenum. *B,* Gastro-intestinal examination. There is a nodular pressure defect on the inner aspect of

(Continued on opposite page.)

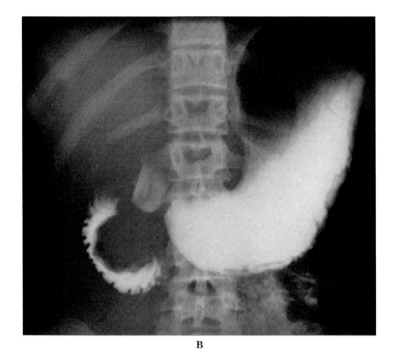

B

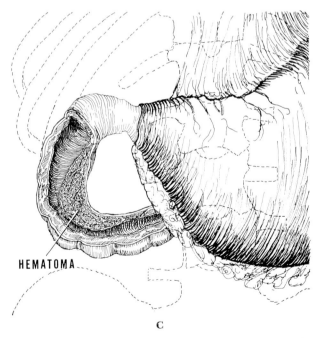

HEMATOMA

C

the duodenal loop. *C*, Diagram. With conservative treatment she made an un-eventful recovery. Gastrointestinal examination 3 months later showed a nor-mal-appearing duodenum.

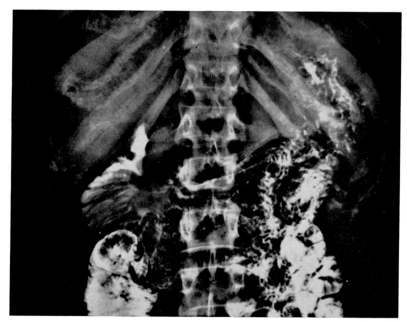

FIGURE 9.3. INTRAMURAL HEMATOMA OF DUODENM; FLATTENING AND WIDENING OF MUCOSAL FOLDS; SPONTANEOUS RECOVERY.

E.F. In an automobile accident, this woman had struck her abdomen against the steering wheel. Barium study shows a pressure defect on the medial aspect of the second portion of the duodenum. The mucosal folds are flattened and the descending duodenum is dilated. With conservative treatment, her symptoms completely subsided.

FLATTENING AND WIDENING OF MUCOSAL FOLDS. Hemorrhage into the wall, particularly the submucosa, causes the mucosal folds to be flattened and widened. This gives the folds a coiled spring appearance (Fig. 9.3).[7]

CONCENTRIC NARROWING. With a more extensive intramural hematoma there is a concentric narrowing of the lumen and effacement of the mucosa (Figs. 9.4 and 9.5). It has not been possible to distinguish intramural hematoma from retroperitoneal periduodenal hemorrhage (Chapter 15), for both produce constriction of the bowel.

Depending on the size of the hematoma, the duodenum may be either completely or partially obstructed. If the obstruction is persistent, surgical intervention is required.[29] Frequently the hematoma is slowly absorbed, releasing the obstruction (Figs. 9.2, 9.3 and 9.5). The patient recovers completely and follow-up radiographs of the duodenum show a return of the caliber and mucosal pattern to normal.

RETROPERITONEAL PERFORATION OF THE DUODENUM. Retroperitoneal perforation is manifest by retroperitoneal air or retroperitoneal hemorrhage.

Retroperitoneal Air. Retroperitoneal emphysema from traumatic

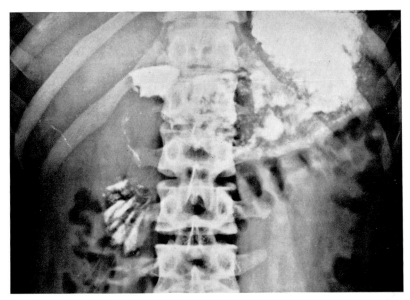

**FIGURE 9.4. INTRAMURAL HEMATOMA OF DUODENUM;
CONSTRICTION OF LUMEN.**

A.I. had a colicky pain following an abdominal injury, then felt better. Within 6 hours he had a recurrence of the pain with nausea and vomiting. Concentric narrowing of the second portion of the duodenum is seen on gastrointestinal examination. At operation, a hematoma in the anterolateral aspect of the descending portion of the duodenum had compressed the muscularis mucosa, causing obstruction.
(Courtesy of L. M. Watanabe, M.D., San Jose Hospital, San Jose, California.)

perforation of the duodenum was first described by Sperling and Rigler[28] in 1937. They noted that intestinal gas dissects into the right perirenal area, along the right psoas muscle, and up under the crus of the diaphragm (Figs. 9.6 and 9.7).

Jacobs, Culver and Koenig[14] point out several additional extensions of retroperitoneal air depending on the location of the duodenal perforation. These are along the root of the transverse mesocolon, along the root of the mesentery of the small bowel, over the right kidney (rarely over the left), downward along the psoas muscle, along the great vessels through the diaphragm into the inferior mediastinum. Although retroperitoneal emphysema is diagnostic when present, it is not a common finding and retroperitoneal perforation can take place without the escape of gas.[3, 10, 16]

Retroperitoneal Hemorrhage. Retroperitoneal hemorrhage from rupture of the duodenum obscures the right kidney and psoas outlines. As the hematoma enlarges, the hepatic flexure of the colon is displaced anteromedially (Fig. 9.8). In this respect, it resembles a perirenal hem-

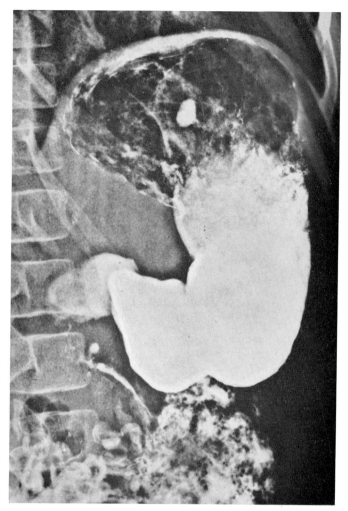

**FIGURE 9.5.   INTRAMURAL HEMATOMA OF DUODENUM;
CONSTRICTION OF LUMEN.**

K.K. had persistent vomiting following abdominal injury. The barium examination shows a marked delay in gastric emptying due to a constriction of the duodenum. At the end of one hour only a small amount of barium had reached the jejunum. Two days later, the barium passed through the constricted area more readily. On conservative treatment, recovery was complete.

(Illustration on opposite page.)

**FIGURE 9.6.   RETROPERITONEAL PERFORATION OF THE THIRD PORTION OF
THE DUODENUM; RIGHT PERIRENAL AIR.**

A, Plain film. R.T. received blows to the abdomen in a fight. On admission continuous abdominal pain and nausea were present. Peritoneal tap revealed old blood clots. Gas outlines the right kidney and extends into the suprarenal area. *B,* Diagram. At operation, a perforated duodenum was found and closed.

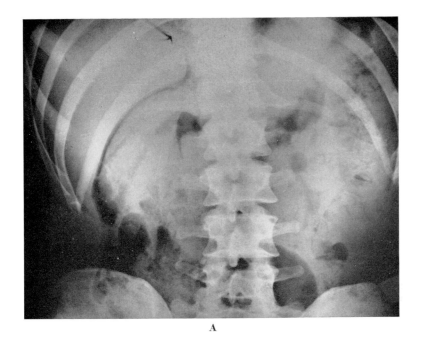

A

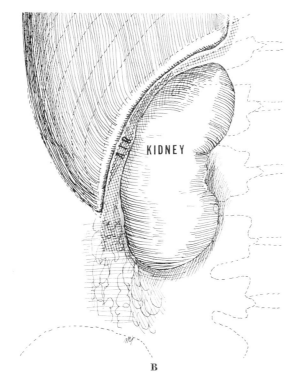

B

Figure 9.6. *Legend on opposite page.*

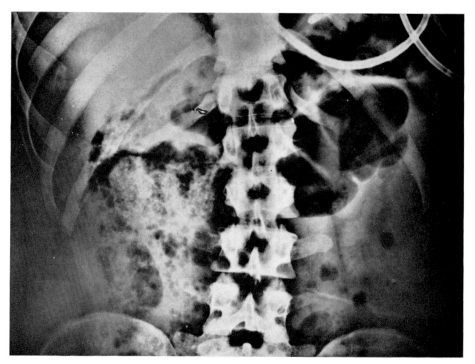

**FIGURE 9.7. RETROPERITONEAL PERFORATION OF THE THIRD PART OF THE
DUODENUM; PERIRENAL AIR.**

R.S. had pain in the lower abdomen radiating into the back after an automobile
accident. There was costovertebral angle tenderness. A large amount of gas
surrounds the right kidney and extends along the right psoas muscle up to the
crus of the diaphragm. The retroperitoneal emphysema was due to rupture of
the third portion of the duodenum.
(Courtesy of George Jacobson, M.D., Los Angeles County Hospital, Los Angeles,
California.)

orrhage. The differentiation is made by means of the intravenous urogram,
which will show both kidneys to function normally when the duodenum
is the site of hemorrhage. Study of the intestinal tract by contrast media
may demonstrate a sinus tract into the retroperitoneal tissues.[26] Retroperitoneal rupture of the duodenum has a high mortality.[24]

Intraperitoneal Rupture

This most commonly occurs in the distal portion of the duodenum at
the ligament of Treitz. Free air is found in the peritoneal cavity, under
the liver or under the diaphragm (Fig. 9.9). There may be fluid and
blood in the peritoneal cavity with widening of the space between the
colon and the fat line. The resultant peritonitis can cause adynamic ileus
of the small and large bowel (Fig. 9.10).

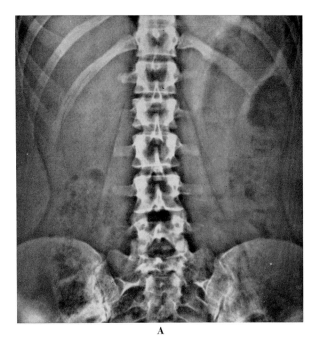

A

FIGURE 9.8. RETROPERI-TONEAL PERFORATION OF DUODENUM; REROPERITO-NEAL HEMORRHAGE.

A, Initial film. In an automobile accident, the seat belt saved this woman from being thrown out, but her abdomen was compressed by the buckle. On admission, the film of the abdomen shows sharply outlined kidneys and psoas muscles. *B,* Twenty-four hour film. Twenty-four hours later, the right kidney and psoas are obscured. The hepatic flexure of the colon is displaced medially and downward. The four quadrant tap was negative. A large right sided retroperitoneal collection of blood was due to a laceration of the duodenum. (Courtesy of Joseph Brozda, M.D., San Jose, California.)

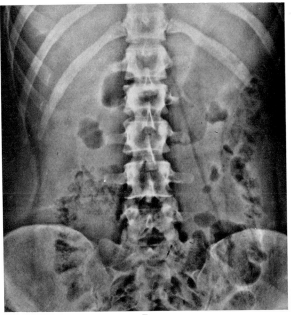

B

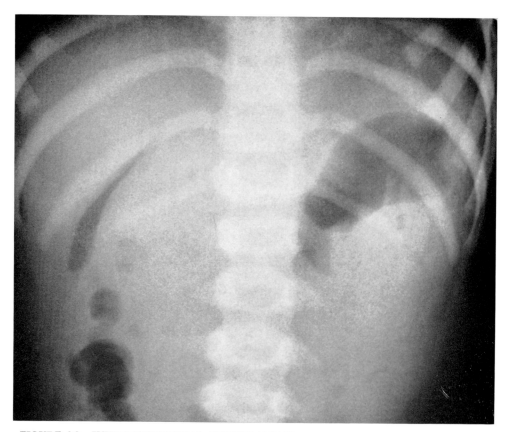

FIGURE 9.9. INTRAPERITONEAL PERFORATION OF THE DUODENUM; FREE AIR.

B.A. This child had vomiting and abdominal distention. Free air is seen along the inferior and lateral aspect of the liver and there is one dilated loop of small bowel in the upper abdomen. The free air was due to a tear in the duodenum 1.5 cm. distal to the pylorus. Hematomas were present in the gastrohepatic ligament and greater omentum.

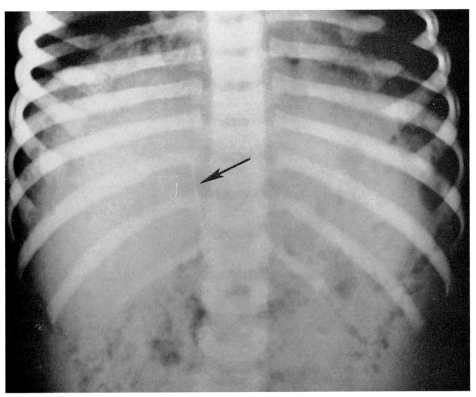

FIGURE 9.10. INTRAPERITONEAL RUPTURE OF THE DUODENUM; GENERALIZED PERITONITIS; FALCIFORM LIGAMENT SIGN.

T.F. This child was vomiting and had difficulty in breathing, multiple contusions and fractures. Numerous small bubbles of gas are present within the abdomen, over the liver and spleen and under the diaphragm. There is air on both sides of the falciform ligament (arrow). The child died, and at autopsy the peritoneum contained 1000 milliliters of yellow turbid fluid from a tear of the duodenum. The father admitted beating the child.

(From McCort, J. J., and Vaudagna, J.: Visceral injuries in battered children. Radiology, 82:424-428, 1964.)

INJURY OF THE JEJUNUM AND ILEUM

Jejunal injury is more common than ileal.[22] In 17 patients with rupture of the small bowel, the jejunum was involved in 13 and the ileum in 4. Rupture of the jejunum occurred close to or within the first twelve inches from the ligament of Treitz; rupture of the ileum occurred close to the ileocecal valve.

Two types of jejunal and ileal injury are found: (1) intramural hematoma, (2) intraperitoneal perforation.

Intramural Hematoma of the Jejunum and Ileum

In a manner similar to that described for the duodenum, hematoma forms in the wall of the small bowel, narrowing the lumen. Radiographically, intramural hematoma in the jejunum appears as an intraluminal mass with widening and flattening of the valvulae conniventes or as an annular constriction. With complete obstruction, operation is required. If the obstruction is incomplete, the patient recovers spontaneously under conservative management.[4, 19]

In patients who have a defect in the clotting mechanism or who are on anticoagulants, multiple intramural hematomas occur spontaneously or as the result of mild trauma.[31]

Intraperitoneal Rupture of the Jejunum and Ileum

Small bowel rupture results from direct contusion of the wall or avulsion of the mesentery.[11]

With rupture of the jejunum or ileum, the majority of patients show evidence of blood and intestinal contents within the peritoneal cavity. *Free intraperitoneal air may be present but is frequently absent in small bowel rupture.*[2] Only 6 of 13 patients with rupture of the jejunum in the author's series had evidence of free air (Fig. 9.11). Occasionally the bowel wall is altered by the presence of hemorrhage and inflammatory exudate. Because of submucosal edema and hemorrhage, the valvulae conniventes are widened, flattened and irregular. The thickened irregular small bowel has a tapered beaklike appearance when the lumen of the bowel is outlined by gas (Figs. 9.12 and 9.13). Proximal to the area of contusion, the small bowel and the stomach are dilated.

Ileal rupture or laceration is less common than jejunal, and was seen in four patients. Only one showed evidence of free air. Two instances were accompanied by fracture of the bony pelvis.

In two patients, the perforation of the small bowel was secondary to

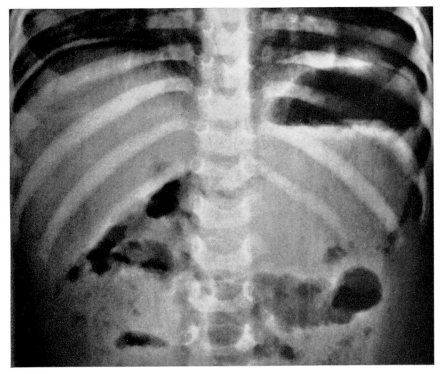

**FIGURE 9.11. PERFORATION OF THE JEJUNUM;
FREE AIR BENEATH THE DIAPHRAGM.**

I.M. had a 3-day history of diarrhea and vomiting. The abdomen was distended, tympanitic and rigid. This film shows a large amount of air beneath the right leaf of the diaphragm. A perforation of the jejunum near the ligament of Treitz was repaired surgically. Trauma was suspected, but no history could be obtained from the parents.

avascular necrosis from tearing of the mesenteric vessels. Initially the radiographic findings were either absent or minimal. There was gradual deterioration of the patient's clinical condition, and the rupture became apparent several days after the injury.

RUPTURE OF THE COLON

Rupture of the colon is also produced by two mechanisms: (1) direct contusion of the bowel wall, (2) avulsion of the mesentery with avascular necrosis[21] (Chapter 8).

When devitalized, the wall of the colon becomes thickened and irregular and the mucosa is ulcerated. Gas in the wall of the bowel is a reliable diagnostic sign of loss of viability[23] (Fig. 9.14). Eventually, the necrotic bowel perforates intra- or retroperitoneally (delayed perforation).

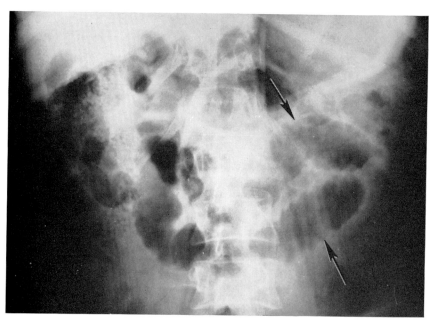

**FIGURE 9.12. PERFORATION OF THE JEJUNUM WITH WIDENING AND
IRREGULARITY OF THE VALVULAE CONNIVENTES.**

J.McG. had abdominal pain following an automobile accident. Free air is
present in the peritoneal cavity and right perirenal area. Air was seen on the
outside of the bowel wall in the right upper quadrant (see Fig. 3.29). One loop
of small bowel has widened, irregular valvulae conniventes (arrows). At operation, a loop of proximal jejunum was found to be lacerated and covered with
fibrinous exudate. Mesenteric contusion was also present.

(Illustration on opposite page.)

**FIGURE 9.13. LACERATION OF THE JEJUNUM AND MESENTERY;
NECROSIS OF THE BOWEL WALL; DELAYED PERFORATION.**

A, Plain film 48 hours after injury. S.A. was struck by the steering wheel.
The small bowel loop in the left abdomen is dilated, and has a thickened and
tapered bowel wall. Signs of intraperitoneal bleeding are present. Air was seen
over the liver in the decubitus projection. *B,* Diagram. At operation, a
mesenteric laceration was found, 2 feet from the ligament of Treitz. The
severed vessels were thrombosed and the bowel supplied by these vessels was
partially necrotic. In addition, the jejunum was perforated transversely along
the mesenteric border.

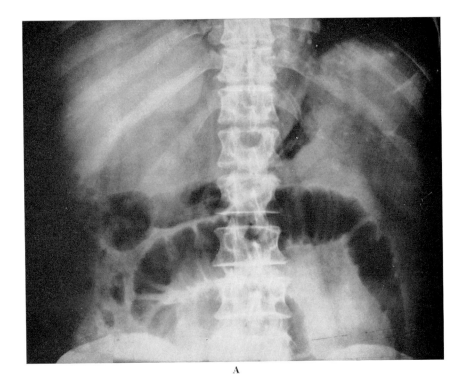

A

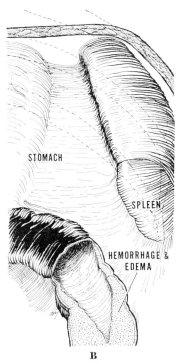

B

Figure 9.13. *See legend on opposite page.*

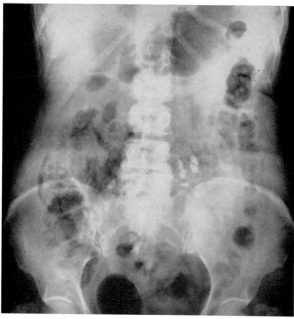

A

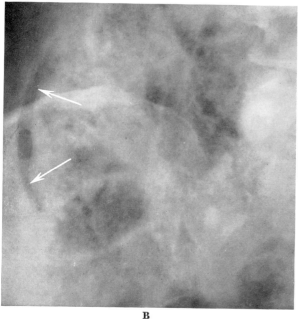

B

FIGURE 9.14. NECROSIS OF CECUM; GAS IN WALL OF BOWEL.

A, Plain film 24 hours after injury. A.D. received a direct blow to the abdomen. This film shows gas and stool within the cecum and ascending colon. *B,* Spot film of cecum. In the lateral wall of the bowel there is a streak of gas (arrows), indicating a break in the continuity of the bowel. Autopsy 24 hours later showed necrosis of the cecum.

(Courtesy of Leo G. Rigler, M.D., University of California, Los Angeles.)

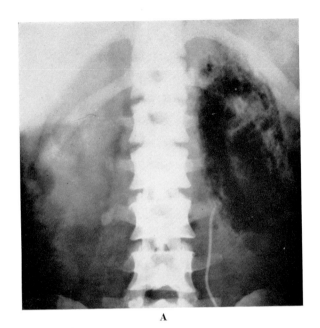

A

FIGURE 9.15. PERFORATION OF THE DESCENDING COLON; LARGE RETROPERITONEAL ABSCESS.

A, Anteroposterior film. F.B., a 35-year-old man, had a separation of the pelvis as well as fractures of the left lower ribs. A mottled collection of gas is seen in the left retroperitoneal area. *B,* Lateral film. The abscess lies posteriorly.

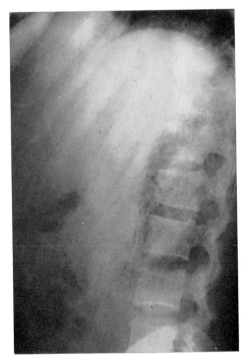

B

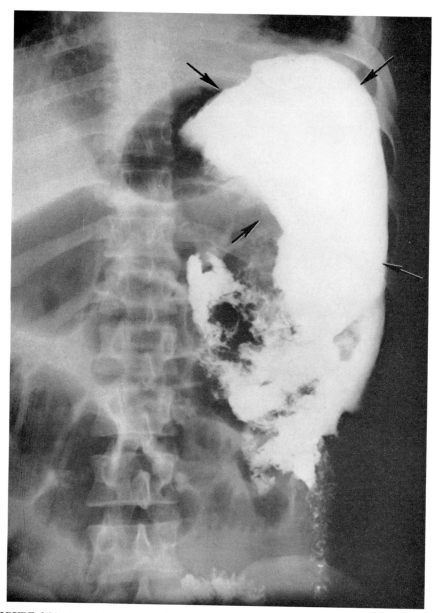

**FIGURE 9.16. DELAYED RETROPERITONEAL PERFORATION OF THE COLON;
ABSCESS CAVITY SHOWN BY BARIUM ENEMA.**

A.S., a 30-year-old man, had been thrown from his car. He had multiple fractures including the left 7th to 12th ribs posteriorly, and a small left pneumothorax. Fifteen days after injury, the patient had pain and was found to have
a localized collection of gas in the left upper abdomen. On enema examination,
the barium enters an abscess cavity in the retroperitoneal tissues through a
colonic perforation (arrows).

Intraperitoneal Rupture of the Colon

The immediate result is peritonitis. On plain film examination, there are gas and stool outside the bowel. The patient is acutely ill and immediate operation is indicated.

Retroperitoneal Rupture of the Colon

A retroperitoneal rupture was found in 4 out of 12 patients with colon injury (Fig. 9.15). The extravasated bowel contents were localized and three of the four patients developed large retroperitoneal abscesses.

Rupture of the Appendix

The appendix is rarely injured in blunt abdominal trauma. An isolated case of traumatic amputation of the appendix has been reported.[9]

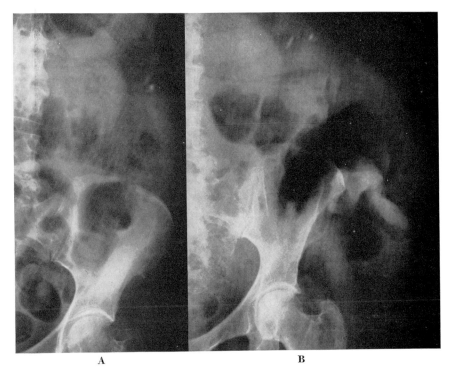

A   B

FIGURE 9.17. DELAYED EXTRAPERITONEAL RUPTURE OF THE DESCENDING COLON; FLANK ABSCESS.

A, Plain film on admission. A.R. sustained multiple rib fractures when struck by an automobile. Six days later she was febrile and was found to have an enlarging left flank mass. *B,* Plain film 4 days later. An accumulation of gas and a soft tissue mass have developed lateral to the left iliac crest. At operation, there was a flank abscess due to an extraperitoneal rupture of the descending colon.

DELAYED RUPTURE OF THE BOWEL

Delayed rupture occurs in both the small intestine and colon (Figs. 9.16 and 9.17). It has been found to follow avascular necrosis of the bowel wall due to interruption of the mesenteric vessels.[6, 11] Hughes and Smaill[12] report an ileal perforation occurring 10 weeks after injury.

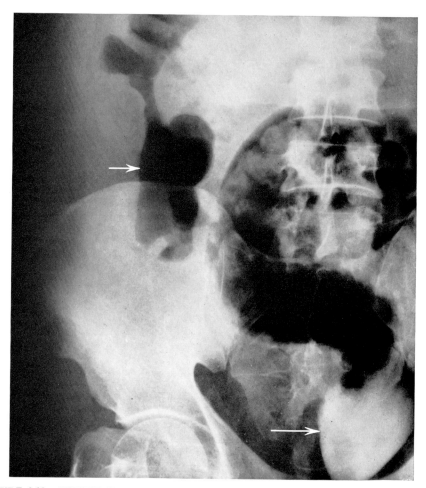

FIGURE 9.18. PERFORATION OF THE CECUM; RIGHT FLANK AND PELVIC ABSCESS.

L.M. This man had been kicked in the right side of the abdomen, and had persistent pain and tenderness. A right flank mass constricts and displaces the ascending colon medially (upper arrow). This mass extends into the pelvis, displacing the bladder to the left side (lower arrow). The fat line on the right is obliterated and the mottled appearance of the mass suggests an abscess. This was due to perforation of the cecum.

ABSCESS FORMATION FROM RUPTURE OF THE BOWEL

Abscess formation follows retroperitoneal rupture of the colon and, occasionally, a retroperitoneal rupture of the duodenum. In one patient with retroperitoneal perforation there was a delay of several weeks following injury before the inflammatory mass appeared (Fig. 9.18).

REFERENCES

1. Albo, R., de Lorimer, A., and Silen, W.: Spontaneous rupture of the stomach in the adult. Surgery, *53*:797-805, 1963.
2. Bosworth, B. M.: Perforation of the small intestine from nonpenetrating abdominal trauma. Amer. J. Surg., *76*:412-422, 1948.
3. Cohn, J., Hawthorne, H. R., and Frobese, A. S.: Retroperitoneal rupture of the duodenum in nonpenetrating abdominal trauma. Amer. J. Surg., *84*:293-301, 1952.
4. Culver, G. J., and Pirson, H. S.: Intramural hematoma of the jejunum. Amer. J. Roentgenol., *90*:732-734, 1963.
5. Davis, D. R., and Thomas, C. Y.: Intramural hematoma of the duodenum and jejunum. A cause of high intestinal obstruction. Report of three cases due to trauma. Ann. Surg., *153*:394-398, 1961.
6. Duncan, J. T.: Rupture of the small intestine through the intact abdominal wall without associated intraperitoneal injury. Amer. Surgeon, *22*:1215-1221, 1956.
7. Felson, B., and Levin, E. J.: Intramural hematoma of duodenum. Radiology, *63*: 823-831, 1951.
8. Ferguson, I. A., and Goode, W. J.: Intramural hematoma of duodenum. Report of a case. New Engl. J. Med., *260*:1176-1177, 1959.
9. Gatewood, J. W., and Russum, W. J.: Injuries to the appendix secondary to blunt trauma. Amer. J. Surg., *91*:558-560, 1956.
10. Gould, R. J., and Thorwarth, W. T.: Retroperitoneal rupture of the duodenum due to blunt nonpenetrating abdominal trauma. Radiology, *80*:743-746, 1963.
11. Hinckley, H. M., and Albertson, H. A.: Avulsion of the mesentery with gangrene of a segment of small bowel (ileum) following non-penetrating trauma of the abdomen. Ann. Surg., *140*:257-259, 1954.
12. Hughes, L. E., and Smaill, G. B.: Long-delayed complications of closed abdominal trauma. Brit. Med. J., *1*:776-777, 1962.
13. Izant, R. J., and Drucker, W. R.: Duodenal obstruction due to intramural hematoma. J. Trauma, *4*:797-818, 1964.
14. Jacobs, E. A., Culver, G. J., and Koenig, E. C.: Roentgenologic aspects of retroperitoneal perforation of the duodenum. Radiology, *43*:563-571, 1944.
15. Jacobson, G., and Carter, R. A.: Small intestinal rupture due to non-penetrating abdominal injury. Amer. J. Roentgenol., *66*:54-64, 1951.
16. Jackson, M. L.: Traumatic retroperitoneal rupture of the duodenum. Amer. J. Surg., *94*:251-256, 1957.
17. Kerry, R. L., and Glas, W. W.: Traumatic injuries of the pancreas and duodenum. Arch. Surg., *85*:813-816, 1962.
18. Kirkpatrick, W. E.: Submucosal hematoma of the duodenum. Discussion and report of a case. Amer. J. Roentgenol., *83*:857-860, 1960.
19. Liverud, K.: Hematoma of jejunum with subileus. Acta Radiol., *30*:163-168, 1948.
20. McCort, J. J., and Vaudagna, J.: Visceral injuries in battered children. Radiology, *82*:424-428, 1964.
21. Penn, I., and Mendels, J.: Gangrene of the caecum following closed abdominal injury. Brit. J. Surg., *50*:112-113, 1962.

22. Poer, D. H., and Woliver, E.: Intestinal and mesenteric injury due to non-penetrating abdominal trauma. J.A.M.A., *118*:11-15, 1942.

23. Rigler, L. G., and Pogue, W. L.: Roentgen signs of intestinal necrosis. Amer. J. Roentgenol., *94*:402-409, 1965.

24. Rothchild, T. P. E., and Hinshaw, J. R.: Retroperitoneal rupture of the duodenum caused by blunt trauma, with a case report. Ann. Surg., *143*:269-275, 1956.

25. Shaw, A., and Cinque, S.: Traumatic intramural hematoma. Amer. J. Dis. Child., *108*:667-673, 1964.

26. Siler, V. E.: Management of rupture of the duodenum due to violence. Amer. J. Surg., *78*:715-728, 1949.

27. Spencer, R., Bateman, J. D., and Horn, P. L.: Intramural hematoma of the intestine, a rare cause of intestinal obstruction. Surgery, *41*:794-804, 1957.

28. Sperling, L., and Rigler, L. G.: Traumatic retroperitoneal rupture of the duodenum. Radiology, *29*:521-524, 1937.

29. Spiro, K.: Retroperitoneal hematoma producing duodenal obstruction. Amer. J. Gastroenterol., *36*:432-434, 1961.

30. Watne, A. L., Butz, G. W., and Tarnay, T. T.: Duodenal obstruction due to intramural hematoma. Arch. Surg., *89*:441-445, 1964.

31. Williams, R. D., and Sargent, F. T.: The mechanism of intestinal injury in trauma. J. Trauma, *3*:289-292, 1963.

32. Wiot, J. F., Weinstein, D. S., and Felson, B.: Duodenal hematoma induced by coumarin. Amer. J. Roentgenol., *86*:70-75, 1961.

10

LACERATION OF THE PANCREAS

CLINICAL OBSERVATIONS

Three mechanisms produce pancreatic injury: (1) a crushing blow to the upper abdomen, (2) a light blow plus acute flexion, (3) sustained and severe flexion of the trunk.[4] The clinical findings depend on the severity of the injury. Traumatic pancreatitis is indicated by an elevated serum amylase and white blood cell count together with midabdominal pain and progressive distention.

Avulsion of the pancreatic vessels causes intra- and retroperitoneal hemorrhage and is manifest clinically by hypovolemic shock.

The value of serial serum amylase determinations in the elucidation of pancreatic injury was initially described by Naffziger and McCorkle[16] in 1943. Numerous other studies have confirmed its usefulness.[2, 6, 18, 21] On the basis of experimental pancreatic injuries in dogs and clinical observations in patients, Nick, Zollinger and Williams[17] have noted that: (1) following blunt trauma, elevation of the serum amylase means pancreatic damage because it is practically never elevated with other gastrointestinal injuries; (2) only a severe blow will injure the pancreas, so that other injuries are commonly associated; (3) in dogs, the serum amylase is uniformly elevated four hours after trauma to the pancreas.

The diagnostic four quadrant tap is said to be most useful in pancreatic injury. A bloody or turbid fluid was aspirated from five of six patients examined by Cleveland et al.[6]

ASSOCIATED INJURIES

Laceration of the liver is a common associated injury and was present in 4 of the author's 13 cases. A periduodenal hematoma was present in 2. Stone et al.[21] found kidney contusion and fractures of spleen and liver as associated injuries.

RADIOGRAPHIC EXAMINATION

Plain Film

The findings on plain film examination of the abdomen in pancreatic trauma are disappointingly meager. In one patient, radiographic changes were completely lacking in the presence of complete transection.

Kinnaird[11] has described gaseous distention of the duodenum and

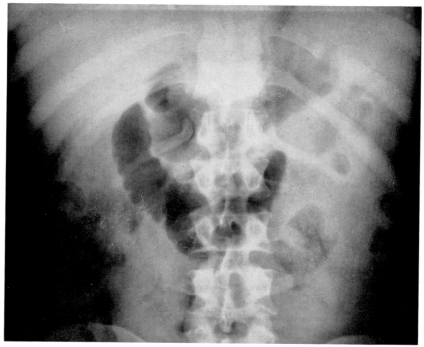

FIGURE 10.1. TRAUMATIC PANCREATITIS. PERSISTENT DILATATION OF THE DUODENUM AND PROXIMAL JEJUNUM (SENTINEL LOOP).

J.P. had been trapped under an automobile. On the following day, dilatation of the duodenum and proximal jejunum is seen. Adynamic ileus of the bowel adjacent to an inflamed pancreas has been called a sentinel loop. It is an uncommon finding in traumatic pancreatitis.

proximal jejunum (sentinel loop). This was found in only 1 of 13 patients studied (Fig. 10.1).

Gastrointestinal Examination

An evaluation of pancreatic injury requires that the stomach and duodenum be opacified by barium sulfate or diatrizoate solution. Retroperitoneal or lesser peritoneal sac hemorrhage displaces the stomach and duodenum forward and may be shown by films taken in the lateral projection.

Selective Arteriography

The use of selective arteriography in acute pancreatic trauma has not been reported. It requires simultaneous catheterization and injection of the celiac axis and the superior mesenteric arteries because both give rise to pancreatic vessels. Pancreatic pseudocysts can be outlined and their nonmalignant nature demonstrated by arteriography (Figs. 10.5 and 10.6).

TYPES OF PANCREATIC INJURY

Two types of pancreatic injury occur: (1) traumatic pancreatitis and (2) pancreatic laceration with hemorrhage.

Traumatic Pancreatitis

This diagnosis is made when, after an accident, the patient has persistent midabdominal pain with elevated serum amylase and white blood cell count. In the experimental study of Anderson and Bergan[1] it was shown that pancreatitis following trauma is dependent on exocrine obstruction and hypersection of the gland.

There are no characteristic radiographic findings.

Conservative treatment by bed rest and antispasmodic and antibiotic medication is favored by some surgeons.[20] Early surgical exploration and drainage is recommended by others.[2, 6, 10, 17]

Laceration of the Pancreas with Bleeding

Depending on the severity of the injury, bleeding takes place in the retroperitoneal space, the lesser peritoneal sac or intraperitoneally.

When the bleeding is limited to the retroperitoneal space around the pancreas, the stomach and duodenum are displaced anteriorly.[9] It is difficult to show such a displacement radiographically.

With concomitant disruption of the gastrocolic mesentery, the blood

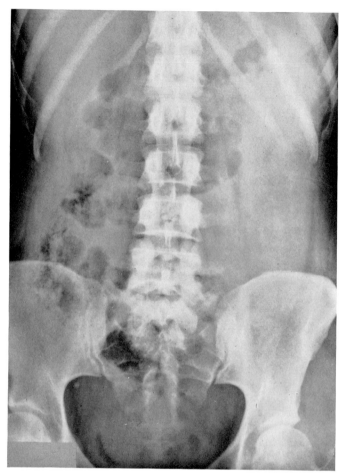

**FIGURE 10.2. LACERATION OF THE PANCREAS;
FREE INTRAPERITONEAL BLEEDING.**

E.J. had evidence of blood in the flanks and pelvis after an automobile accident. No operation was performed. She died suddenly 5 days later. Autopsy showed intra-abdominal hemorrhage with peritonitis, due to a laceration of the head of the pancreas and acute hemorrhagic pancreatitis.

(Courtesy of George Hoeffler, M.D., Community Hospital of San Mateo County, San Mateo, California.)

from the torn pancreas enters the peritoneal cavity to fill the pelvis and flanks (Fig. 10.2). Unless other findings are present, such as displacement of the stomach and duodenum, there is no way of identifying the origin of this blood.

TRAUMATIC PSEUDOCYST

With disruption of the pancreatic ducts, pancreatic secretions accumulate in the retroperitoneal tissues, forming a pseudocyst.[13, 14] This does not have a mucous membrane lining and is covered by either the peritoneum of the pancreas or the serosa of adjacent organs.[12] In the adult, pseudocyst usually results from infection.[5, 19] In infants and children, it usually follows trauma.[8, 15] Pseudocyst may form very rapidly; in one patient a cyst appeared within one week after injury (Fig. 10.4).

Depending on its location, the cyst will displace the stomach superiorly, inferiorly or anteriorly. Anterior displacement is most common. Characteristically, the cyst is round and smooth in outline. Where the cyst impinges on the stomach and duodenum, the mucosal folds are flattened. At the site of impingement, the gastric and duodenal wall has a double contour (Fig. 10.6). Within a short time, it may reach a very large size (Fig. 10.4). On arteriography, the pancreatic vessels are elongated and attenuated by the swelling of the cyst. There is an absence of tumor vessels (Figs. 10.5 and 10.6).

COMPLICATIONS OF PANCREATIC LACERATION

Sterile Pleural Effusion

A left-sided pleural effusion may follow traumatic pancreatitis or a laceration of the pancreas (Fig. 10.7). On aspiration, this fluid is sterile and shows a high amylase content. Usually, the pleural effusion will regress when the pancreatic injury is repaired.[3]

Pancreatic Abscess

Pancreatic abscesses may complicate injury to the pancreas when there is a large undrained collection of pancreatic secretion and blood in the surrounding tissues.[7] Pathogenic bacteria presumably enter by way of the blood stream. These abscesses can extend into the lesser sac or beneath the left leaf of the diaphragm (Fig. 10.8).

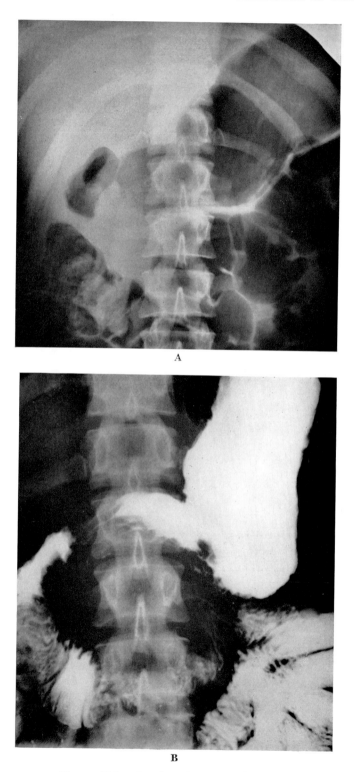

A

B

Figure 10.3. *Continued on opposite page.*

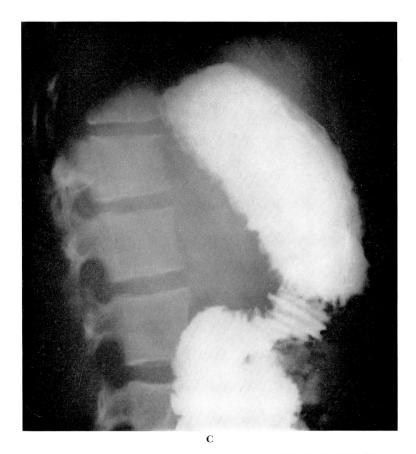

C

FIGURE 10.3. TRAUMATIC PSEUDOCYST OF THE PANCREAS.

A, Plain film, third day. L.W. had been injured in an automobile accident. On the third hospital day, her serum amylase was 432 Somogyi units, and the plain film of the abdomen shows a density overlying the gas-filled duodenum and distal stomach. At operation, there was a 6 cm. laceration of the left lobe of the liver and marked hemorrhage about the head of the pancreas. *B,* Gastrointestinal series, fourteenth day, AP films. Two weeks later, the patient developed a mass in the midabdomen. The barium examination shows a widening of the duodenal loop with evidence of extrinsic pressure on the distal stomach and the third portion of the duodenum. *C,* Gastrointestinal series, fourteenth day, lateral films. The duodenum is displaced anteriorly. At re-operation, a 10 cm. cyst of the head of the pancreas was drained.
(Courtesy of William Thompson, M.D., Peninsula Hospital, Burlingame, California.)

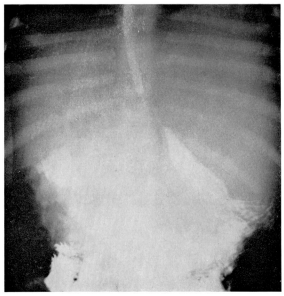

A

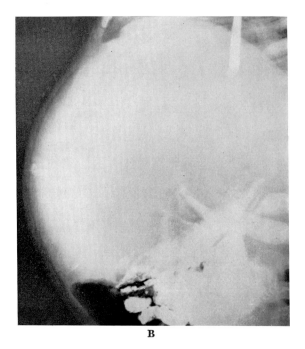

B

FIGURE 10.4. POST-TRAUMATIC PSEUDOCYST OF THE PANCREAS; DISPLACEMENT OF THE STOMACH AND SMALL BOWEL.

A, Gastrointestinal series, AP film. C.P. had been run over by an automobile. One week after injury, the abdomen became distended and the child vomited repeatedly. *B,* Gastrointestinal series, lateral film. The mass is found to displace the barium-filled stomach and small bowel posteriorly and inferiorly. At operation, a thin-walled cyst was found to arise from the pancreas and fill the entire upper abdomen.

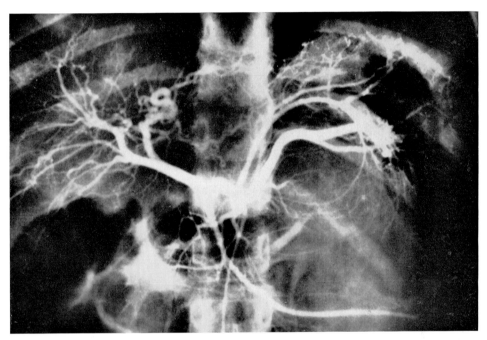

**FIGURE 10.5. TRAUMATIC PSEUDOCYST OF THE PANCREAS;
SELECTIVE ARTERIOGRAPHY.**

H.O.C. This patient developed a left upper quadrant mass following abdominal injury. By retrograde femoral approach the tip of the catheter was placed in the celiac axis. In the arterial phase, the mass is avascular and the major arteries supplying the pancreas are elongated and attenuated. No peripheral tumor type vessels are seen.

(Courtesy of Tord Olin, M.D., Lund, Sweden.)

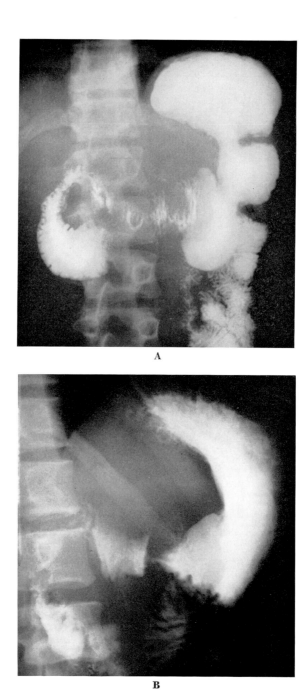

A

B

**FIGURE 10.6. TRAUMATIC PSEUDOCYST OF THE PANCREAS; FLATTENING OF MU-
COSAL FOLDS; DOUBLE CONTOUR OF STOMACH CAUSED BY EXTRINSIC PRESSURE.**

A, Gastrointestinal series, AP films. J.A., a 23-year-old man, sustained abdominal
injury in a fight. He had severe abdominal pain, vomiting and an elevated serum

(*Continued on opposite page.*)

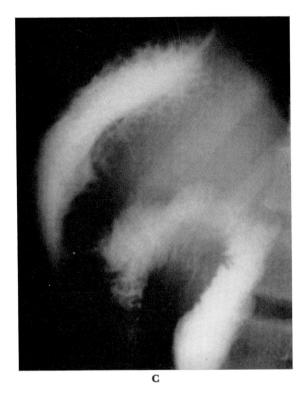

C

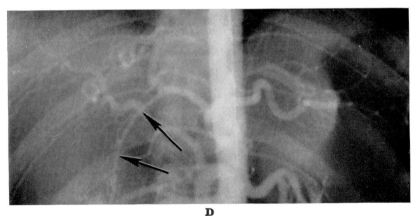

D

amylase. Three days later, a mass was palpable in the upper abdomen. On the posteroanterior film of the upper G.I. series, the mucosal folds in the distal stomach are compressed but not thickened. *B,* Gastrointestinal series, right anterior oblique. The oblique film shows a mass displacing the stomach anteriorly. The mass is smooth, and a double contour of the stomach is formed, indicating that the mass is extrinsic. *C,* Gastrointestinal series, right lateral. The right lateral film of the abdomen confirms the retrogastric position of the mass. *D,* Arteriogram. A catheter was placed in the abdominal aorta by a retrograde femoral approach. The gastroduodenal artery (arrow) is elongated and stretched by the mass.

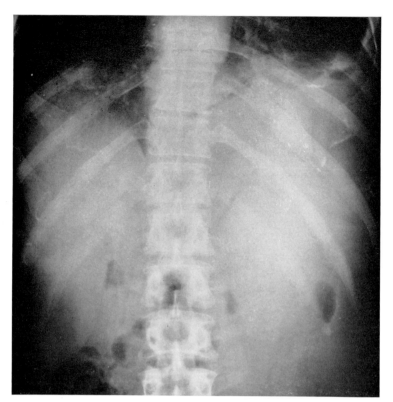

FIGURE 10.7. TRAUMATIC PSEUDOCYST OF THE PANCREAS; LEFT PLEURAL EFFUSION.

M.H. had fallen and had struck the left lower rib cage. On this film, 17 days later, fluid is present in the left pleural space. A soft tissue mass fills the entire left upper quadrant, displacing the splenic flexure downward and the body of the stomach medially. There is no sign of intraperitoneal bleeding. The mass, a large indurated and inflamed cyst, filled the lesser omental sac and adhered to the diaphragm and posterior peritoneum.

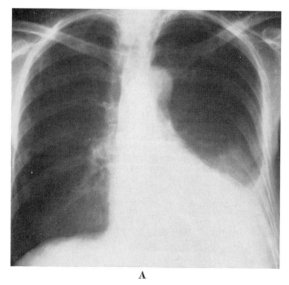

A

Figure 10.8. *Continued on opposite page.*

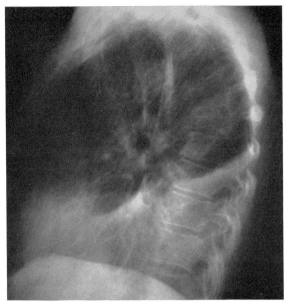

B

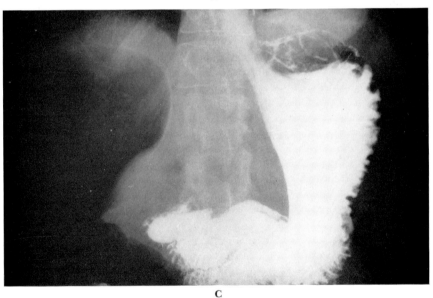

C

**FIGURE 108. SEQUELAE OF A TRAUMATIC PANCREATITIS;
LEFT SUBDIAPHRAGMATIC ABSCESS AND PLEURAL EFFUSION.**

A, Posteroanterior chest film. F.R. had fractures of the right 8th and 11th ribs and the left 5th to 7th ribs, with compression fractures of T4 and T7. At subsequent laparotomy, a laceration of the liver was repaired and the spleen was removed. Postoperatively, fluid with a high amylase content drained from the incision. *B,* Right lateral chest film. Eight months later, acute abdominal pain developed after the drainage had ceased. The serum amylase was 561 Somogyi units. The chest x-ray reveals left pleural effusion. On aspiration, it had an amylase content of 548 Somogyi units and was sterile. *C,* Upright abdomen after pneumoperitoneography. N_2O did not dissect beneath the left leaf of the diaphragm because of inflammatory adhesions. A mass presents between the gastric fundus and the diaphragm. A left subdiaphragmatic abscess was drained.

157

REFERENCES

1. Anderson, M. C., and Bergan, J. J.: An experimental study of pancreatic trauma and its relationship to pancreatic inflammation. Arch. Surg., 86:1044-1050, 1963.
2. Baker, R. J., Dippel, W. F., Freeark, R. J., and Strohl, E. L.: The surgical significance of trauma to the pancreas. Arch. Surg., 86:1038-1044, 1963.
3. Bickford, B. J.: Traumatic pseudo-cyst of the pancreas with pleural effusion. Brit. Med. J. 1:1134-1135, 1948.
4. Bracey, D. W.: Complete rupture of the pancreas. Brit. J. Surg., 48:575-576, 1961.
5. Brilhart, K. B., and Priestly, J. T.: Pseudocysts of pancreas. Amer. J. Surg., 81: 151-160, 1951.
6. Cleveland, H. C., Reinschmidt, J. S., and Waddell, W. R.: Traumatic pancreatitis, an increasing problem. Surg. Clin. North America, 43:401-411, 1963.
7. Culotta, R. J., Howard, J. M., and Jordan, G. L.: Traumatic injuries of pancreas. Surgery, 40:320-327, 1956.
8. Di Censo, S., Ginsberg, S. B., and Snyder, W. H.: Pancreatic pseudocysts in childhood. Surg. Gynec. Obstet., 119:1049-1052, 1964.
9. Estes, W. L., Bowman, T. L., and Melicke, F. F.: Non-penetrating abdominal trauma with special reference to lesions of the duodenum and pancreas. Amer. J. Surg., 83:434-446, 1952.
10. Joseph, M.: Pancreas and the steering wheel. Western J. Surg., 60:129-131, 1952.
11. Kinnaird, P. W.: Pancreatic injuries due to non-penetrating abdominal trauma. Amer. J. Surg., 91:552-557, 1956.
12. Knopf, H.: Traumatic bursa-omentalis cyst. Zentralbl. Chir., 78:1997-1918, 1953.
13. Letton, R. H., and Wilson, J. P.: Traumatic severance of pancreas treated by roux-Y anastomosis. Surg. Gynec. Obstet., 109:473-478, 1959.
14. Mathewson, C., and Halter, B. L.: Traumatic pancreatitis. Amer. J. Surg., 83:409-442, 1952.
15. Miller, R. E.: Pancreatic pseudocysts in infants and children. Arch. Surg., 89:517-521, 1964.
16. Naffziger, H. C., and McCorkle, H. J.: The recognition and management of acute trauma to the pancreas: With particular reference to the use of the serum amylase test. Ann. Surg., 118:594-602, 1943.
17. Nick, W. V., Zollinger, R. W., and Williams, R. D.: The diagnosis of traumatic pancreatitis with blunt abdominal injuries. J. Trauma, 5:495-502, 1965.
18. Phillips, S. K., and Seybold, W. D.: Traumatic rupture of pancreas. Proc. Mayo Clin., 23:254-260, 1948.
19. Pinkham, R. D.: Pancreatic collections (pseudocysts) following pancreatitis and pancreatic necrosis. Surg. Gynec. Obstet., 80:225-235, 1945.
20. Rini, J.: Traumatic pancreatitis. Amer. Surgeon, 18:596-601, 1952.
21. Stone, H. H., Stowens, K. B., and Shipley, S. H.: Injuries to the pancreas. Arch. Surg., 85:525-530, 1962.

11

LACERATION OF THE DIAPHRAGM

CLINICAL OBSERVATIONS

Approximately 95 per cent of tears involve the left leaf of the diaphragm.[4, 12] A tear in both leaves of the diaphragm is exceedingly rare and usually is fatal.[18, 19, 21] Because the diaphragm is the major muscle of respiration, serious injury is immediately manifest by rapid and labored breathing. Herniation of the abdominal viscera into the thorax shifts the mediastinal structures to the opposite side and displaces the apical impulse and heart sounds. The combination of collapsed lung and intrathoracic bleeding is indicated by absent breath sounds and dullness to percussion. With extensive damage to the diaphragm and concomitant bleeding, shock supervenes. Immediate surgical repair of diaphragmatic rupture is indicated.[25]

ASSOCIATED INJURIES

The diaphragmatic muscle is liable to tear and rupture when the abdomen is subject to a sudden increase in pressure. In the patients seen at the Santa Clara County Hospital, rupture of the diaphragm rarely occurred alone, but almost always in association with injury to adjacent viscera. Of 20 patients with diaphragmatic ruptures reported by Grage et al.,[16] 18 had injury to other organs. Uncomplicated rupture of the diaphragm has a good prognosis, but the outlook worsens in relation to the severity

159

of associated injuries.[26] Lucido and Wall[18] found the spleen to be injured in 21 of 47 patients with diaphragmatic rupture. Other accompanying injuries are fracture of the ribs and pelvis, and laceration of the liver or kidney.[1, 2] When a crushing abdominal injury is the cause of diaphragmatic tear, an associated pelvic fracture is likely to be found.[8, 14, 16]

TECHNIQUE OF EXAMINATION OF THE DIAPHRAGM

Chest Radiography

Because rupture of the spleen and pelvic fracture are often accompanied by injury to the diaphragm, a chest radiograph is obtained on all patients with abdominal injury. The patient with diaphragmatic injury is often in

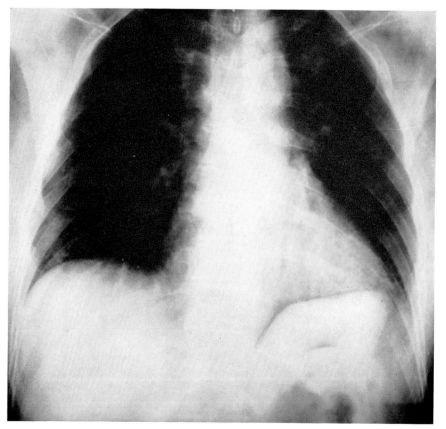

**FIGURE 11.1.   IRREGULARITY OF THE LEFT HEMIDIAPHRAGM;
AN EARLY SIGN OF INJURY.**

M.A.V. sustained severe contusions in an automobile accident. This film, on admission, shows an alteration in the normal convex outline of the left hemidiaphragm with a small amount of fluid in the left pleural space. Thirty-seven days later the diaphragm suddenly ruptured with herniation of the stomach, small intestine and spleen into the left thorax.

respiratory distress and is breathing rapidly. Consequently, the exposure time must be reduced as low as possible to obtain satisfactory radiographs. Loss of sharpness of the diaphragm or any asymmetry of the diaphragm calls for further studies (Fig. 11.1). Fluid in the pleural space indicates possible diaphragmatic tear. If the diaphragm is obscured by intrapleural blood, it can be unmasked by placing the patient in the opposite lateral decubitus position and using a horizontal beam. Four roentgen signs of traumatic diaphragmatic hernia are described by Carter, Giuseffi and Felson:[9] (1) an archlike shadow resembling an abnormally high diaphragm; (2) gas bubbles, homogeneous densities or other abnormal markings extending above the anticipated level of the normal diaphragm; (3) shift of the heart and mediastinal structures (frequently present and dependent on the volume of viscera and fluid encroaching on the thoracic space; (4) disc or platelike atelectasis in the lung base.

Fluoroscopy of the Diaphragm

Fluoroscopy of the diaphragm is employed in questionable cases. When both leaves move downward on inspiration freely and equally, injury is unlikely. Any alteration in position or mobility of the diaphragm is suspicious and calls for careful follow-up study by repeated fluoroscopy and serial roentgenography to detect delayed rupture and herniation.

Barium Swallow and Enema

When herniation of the abdominal viscera into the thorax is suspected, the stomach, small bowel or colon is opacified (Figs. 11.2 and 11.4). An abnormal position of the nasogastric tube also indicates herniation of the stomach (Fig. 11.5).

Pneumoperitoneography

If the diaphragm cannot be clearly delineated, a small pneumoperitoneum is useful. Usually 50 milliliters of 100 per cent carbon dioxide is sufficient to outline the undersurface of the diaphragm. If a rent is present in the diaphragm, the carbon dioxide will enter the thorax and produce a small pneumothorax. This amount of gas in the pleural space will not significantly reduce the respiratory capacity and is readily absorbed from both the peritoneum and pleura.

TYPES OF DIAPHRAGMATIC INJURY

Left Leaf Rupture

When the left leaf ruptures, adjacent abdominal organs enter the thorax. Most commonly the stomach, the splenic flexure of the colon, the

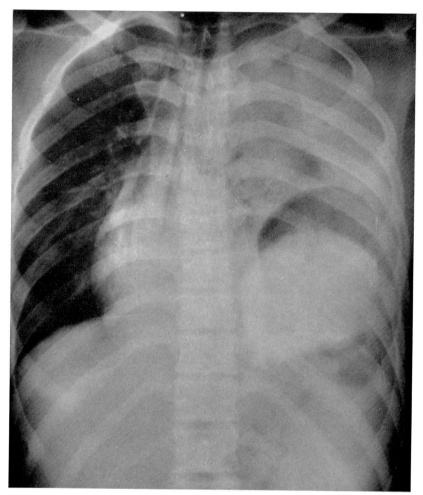

FIGURE 11.2. RUPTURE OF THE LEFT HEMIDIAPHRAGM; HERNIATION OF STOMACH, COLON AND LIVER; HEMOTHORAX.

Following an automobile accident, J.L. had left chest pain. There is marked shift of the mediastinum to the right, with blood in the right pleural space. The stomach, opacified by barium sulfate, is in the left thorax. A splenic mass displaces the colon medially. At operation, the left pleural cavity was filled with blood. The stomach, transverse colon and left lobe of the liver herniated through a stellate diaphragmatic tear. The spleen was ruptured.
(Courtesy of Stanford Rossiter, M.D., Sequoia Hospital, Redwood City, California.)

small bowel, the spleen and the omentum will herniate. The presence of a gas-filled stomach, small bowel or colon in the left thorax is diagnostic (Figs. 11.2, 11.3 and 11.4). The radiologist can confirm the diagnosis by introducing diatrizoate sodium or barium sulfate into the stomach. If these substances will not enter the stomach, incarceration of the hernia is likely. Failure of the barium given by enema to pass into the herniated

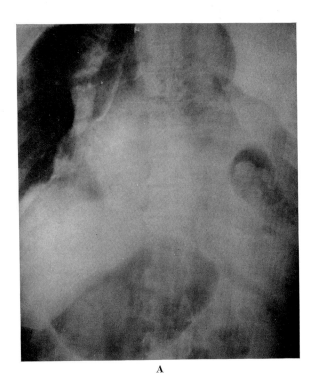

A

FIGURE 11.3. RUPTURE OF THE LEFT HEMIDIA-PHRAGM; RUPTURE OF THE SPLEEN; HERNIATION OF THE COLON; FRACTURES OF THE LEFT RIBS.

A, Anteroposterior film of thorax and upper abdomen. S.D. was admitted with severe shock and respiratory difficulty following injury. The colon is present within the left thorax. The left lung is compressed and the mediastinal structures are displaced to the right. *B,* Diagram. Blood fills the left pleural space and peritoneal cavity.

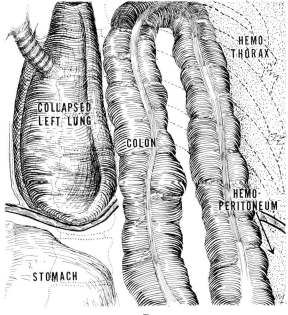

B

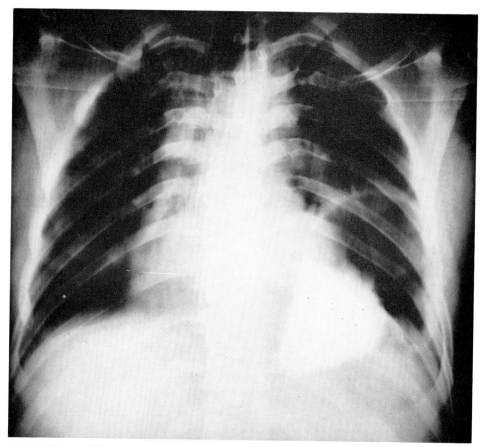

FIGURE 11.4. RUPTURE OF LEFT HEMIDIAPHRAGM; STOMACH IN LEFT THORAX.
R.G. suffered multiple fractures and contusions in an automobile accident. On admission, the stomach bubble was found in the left chest. This was confirmed by instilling barium sulfate through a nasogastric tube.

large bowel also indicates incarceration.[9, 23] With herniation and incarceration, the blood supply of the viscera may be compromised and immediate surgical repair is indicated.[5, 6] When the abdominal viscera extend into the left thorax, marked compression of the left lung occurs with a shift of the mediastinum to the right side (Fig. 11.6). Reduced respiratory reserve causes dyspnea. When the tear of the diaphragm is associated with avulsion of the vascular pedicle of the spleen, bleeding is profuse and a large amount of blood collects in the pleural and peritoneal spaces (Figs. 11.2 and 11.3).

Occasionally, when the wall of the gastric fundus is entirely within the left thorax it will mimic a high diaphragm (Fig. 11.6).[15] Insertion of a nasogastric tube or administration of barium or diatrizoate enables the radiologist to avoid this error (Figs. 11.2, 11.4 and 11.5).

Right Leaf Rupture

With rupture of the right leaf of the diaphragm there may be a herniation of the liver, and, less frequently, other intra-abdominal organs, usually the small bowel.[22, 24] A split in the muscle occurs most commonly in the anteromedial aspect.[13] Radiographically, a gas-filled loop of bowel in the right thorax is diagnostic. Most commonly, the liver alone herniates into the thorax and the herniated liver must be differentiated from a high, paralyzed right leaf of the diaphragm of infrapulmonary effusion (Fig. 11.7). In the right lateral decubitis projection of the chest, an infra-

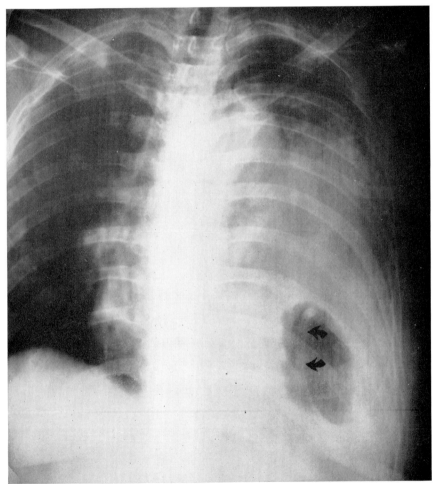

FIGURE 11.5. RUPTURE OF LEFT HEMIDIAPHRAGM; HERNIATION OF STOMACH SHOWN BY POSITION OF NASOGASTRIC TUBE.

E.R. was pinned under her car and suffered fractures of the left 2nd to 4th ribs. The presence of gastric folds and the tip of the nasogastric tube (arrows) within the gas bubble in the left thorax shows that this is a herniated stomach. Blood is present in the left thorax.

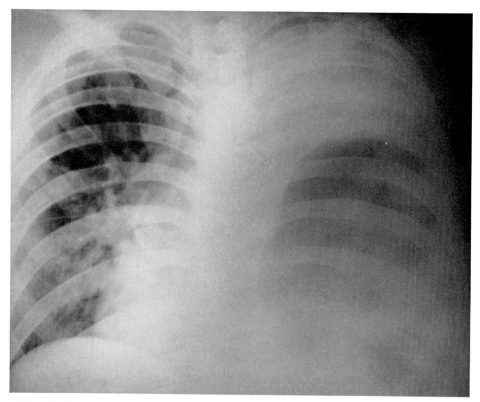

FIGURE 11.6. RUPTURE OF LEFT HEMIDIAPHRAGM; HERNIATION OF STOMACH.

J.M. had continuous abdominal pain following an automobile accident in which he sustained a fractured pelvis and contused bladder. The convexity of the superior margin of the gas in the left thorax indicates that it is contained within a dilated herniated stomach.

pulmonary effusion will gravitate into the lateral thorax. With a paralyzed diaphragm or with herniation, the liver edge is high in position. Liver herniation is said to simulate an intrathoracic tumor.[10]

Pneumoperitoneography is a valuable diagnostic aid.[11] A small amount of gas introduced into the abdomen passes into the right pleural space unless the liver is incarcerated. The presence of a small pneumothorax is conclusive (Fig. 11.7).

DELAYED RUPTURE OF THE DIAPHRAGM

Delayed rupture is not uncommon.[28] The diaphragm may appear normal in the admission radiograph. Within a few days, the patient may develop dyspnea and shock with flat percussion tone and diminished breath sounds. Radiography and fluoroscopy confirm a delayed rupture with herniation (Figs. 11.8 and 11.9). An asymptomatic interval of six weeks following initial injury occurred in one of the author's patients. A strangulated Richter's hernia of the stomach through a rent in the diaphragm from injury three years earlier was reported by Arndt et al.[3] Carter et al.[9] found that 90 per cent of strangulated diaphragmatic hernias were traumatic in origin, and 85 per cent occurred within three years of injury. Strangulation was noted as late as 10 years after injury. In a study of 500 patients who had a surgical repair of hiatus hernia, Lortat-Jacob et al.[17] found that 14 had a history of serious trauma. They believe that hiatus hernia can follow acute thoraco-abdominal injury.

TRAUMATIC WEAKENING OF THE DIAPHRAGM (EVENTRATION)

Following an injury to the diaphragm, traumatic necrosis may cause a loss of muscle tissue. The injured muscle is replaced by fibrous tissue, which is less strong and efficient than the contralateral leaf. After a variable time interval, the traumatized and atrophic diaphragm occupies a position higher than the normal.[20] It will move downward on inspiration, but with less amplitude and vigor than the normal side (Fig. 11.10). This inequality of diaphragmatic motion is readily apparent on fluoroscopy and is magnified by having the patient sniff on inspiration. A traumatized and weakened diaphragm can be differentiated fluoroscopically from a paralyzed diaphragm, which moves in a paradoxical manner—"Kienboch's sign."[27]

Recurrent lower lobe pneumonia may occur on the involved side due to respiratory inefficiency.[7]

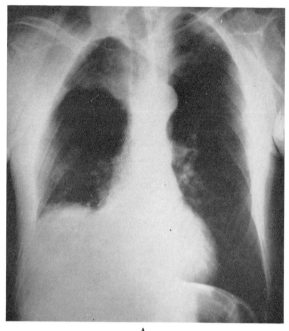

A

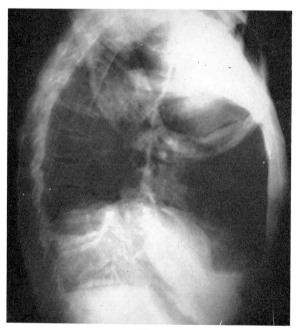

B

FIGURE 11.7. RUPTURE OF THE RIGHT HEMIDIAPHRAGM; HERNIATION OF THE LIVER; DEMONSTRATION BY SMALL CARBON DIOXIDE PNEUMOPERITONEUM.

A, Preliminary chest film, posteroanterior. *B,* Lateral. J.C. had fractures of the extremities, but no complaints referable to his chest. Two days following ad-

(Continued on opposite page.)

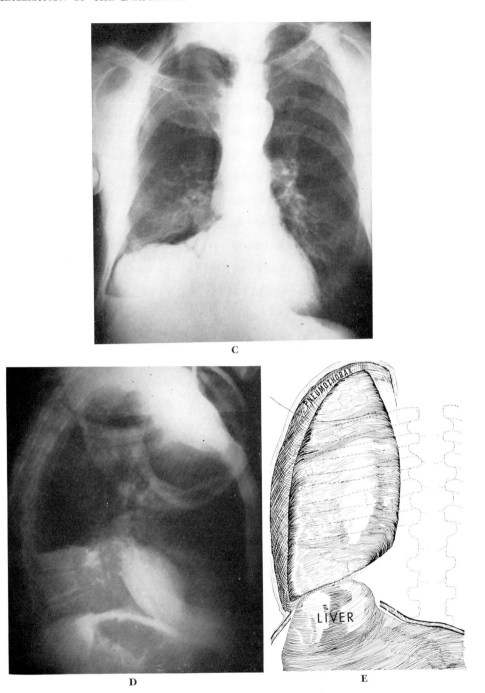

C

D   E

mission, the right leaf of the diaphragm was found to be elevated and irregular, with plate atelectasis at the right lung base. On the abdominal film, the hepatic flexure was high in position and the inferior border of the liver could not be identified. *C,* Chest film after pneumoperitoneography, posteroanterior. *D,* Lateral. A small pneumoperitoneum, using carbon dioxide, shows the gas in the right pleural space. *E,* Diagram. At operation, the liver was projecting into the right thoracic cavity through a defect in the diaphragm.

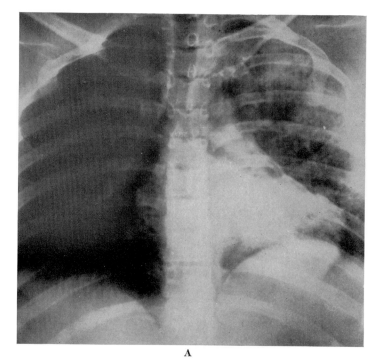

A

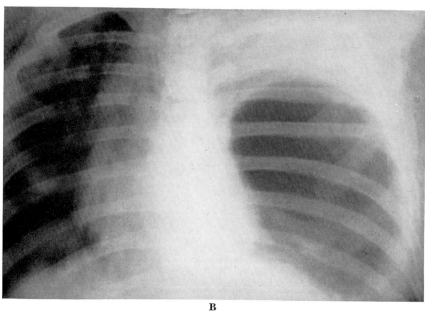

B

FIGURE 11.8. DELAYED RUPTURE OF THE LEFT HEMIDIAPHRAGM (TWO DAYS).

A, Initial chest film. G.M.C. Following an automobile accident, this girl had a cerebral concussion, fracture-dislocation of C2, fracture of the pelvis and multiple left rib fractures. Initial film of the chest shows slight elevation of the left leaf of the diaphragm, with contusion of the left lung. *B,* Chest film at 48 hours. The gas-filled stomach has entered the left thorax, with marked compression of the left lung and displacement of the mediastinal structures to the right side.

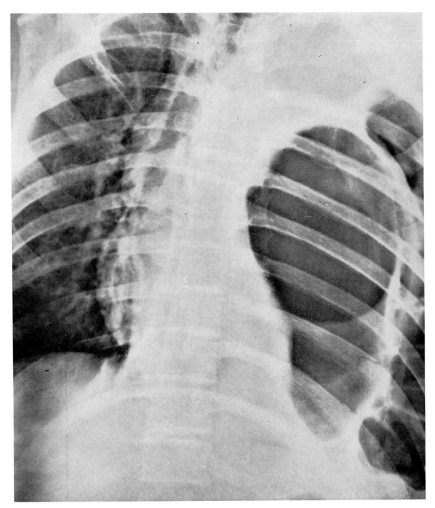

**FIGURE 11.9. DELAYED RUPTURE OF THE LEFT HEMIDIAPHRAGM;
HERNIATION OF THE COLON AND STOMACH.**

R.S. had multiple contusions and lacerations and fractures of the left 9th and
10th ribs. On the initial film, the lungs were clear and both leaves of the diaphragm intact. Two days later complete rupture of the left leaf of the diaphragm
is found with the stomach and colon in the left thorax. The left lung is compressed and the mediastinum shifted to the right. A complete tear of the
diaphragm from the lateral chest wall was found.
(Courtesy of Stanford Rossiter, M.D., Sequoia Hospital, Redwood City,
California.)

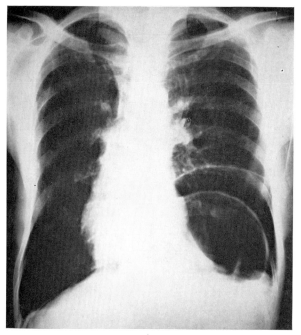

A

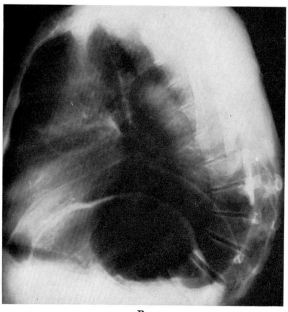

B

**FIGURE 11.10. POST-TRAU-
MATIC HIGH, THIN DIA-
PHRAGM; PNEUMOPERI-
TONEOGRAPHY.**

A, Posteroanterior upright
film. B.F. injured the left
hemidiaphragm in a train
accident in 1933. *B,* Lateral upright film. Twen-
ty-four years later, the
diaphragm is found, by
pneumoperitoneography, to
be very thin. This finding
was confirmed subsequently
when he had a laparotomy
for an unrelated duodenal
ulcer.

REFERENCES

1. Adams, T. W., and Musselman, M. M.: Recognition and management of the triad of injury to the spleen, kidney and diaphragm. Amer. J. Surg., 87:452-456, 1954.
2. Alivisatos, C. N., Bonellos, C. H., Avlamis, G. P., Sarris, M. C., and Romanos, A. N.: Traumatic closed rupture of the diaphragm. Dis. Chest, 46:435-440, 1964.
3. Arndt, J. H., Healy, M. J., and Schonfeld, M. D.: Strangulated Richter's hernia of the stomach. Amer. J. Roentgenol., 91:766-769, 1964.
4. Bartley, O., and Wickbom, I.: Roentgenologic diagnosis of rupture of the diaphragm. Acta Radiol., 53:33-41, 1960.
5. Bernatz, P. E., Burnside, A. F., and Clagett, O. T.: Problems of ruptured diaphragm. J.A.M.A., 168:877-881, 1958.
6. Blades, B.: Traumatic diaphragmatic hernia. Amer. J. Surg., 105:501-504, 1963.
7. Bohrer, S. P.: X-Ray Seminar. No. 22. Recurrent right lower lobe disease. J.A.M.A. 184:229-231, 1963.
8. Carlson, R. I., Diveley, W. L., Gobbel, W. G., and Daniel, R. A.: Dehiscence of the diaphragm associated with fractures of the pelvis or lumbar spine due to nonpenetrating wounds of the chest and abdomen. J. Thorac. Cardiov. Surg., 36:254-261, 1958.
9. Carter, B. N., Giuseffi, J., and Felson, B.: Traumatic diaphragmatic hernia. Amer. J. Roentgenol., 65:56-72, 1951.
10. Child, C., Haram, G. S., Dotter, C. T., and Steinberg, I.: Liver herniation simulating intrathoracic tumor. J. Thorac. Cardiov. Surg., 21:391-393, 1951.
11. Clay, R. C., and Hanlon, C. R.: Pneumoperitoneum in the differential diagnosis of diaphragmatic hernia. J. Thorac. Cardiov. Surg., 21:57-70, 1957.
12. Desforges, G., Streider, J. W., Lynch, J. P., and Madoff, I. M.: Traumatic rupture of the diaphragm. J. Thorac. Cardiov. Surg., 34:779-804, 1957.
13. Dugan, D. J., and Merrill, D. L.: Right phrenohepatic incarceration. Amer. J. Surg., 94:208-217, 1957.
14. Evans, C. J., and Simpson, J. A.: Fifty-seven cases of diaphragmatic hernia and eventration. Thorax, 5:343-361, 1950.
15. Fawcett, A. W., and Des, J. B.: Diaphragmatic hernia due to blunt trauma. Lancet, 1:662-664, 1958.
16. Grage, T., McLean, L., and Campbell, G.: Traumatic rupture of the diaphragm Surgery, 46:669-681, 1959.
17. Lortat-Jacob, J. L., Clot, J. P., and Fekete, F.: Hernies hiatales et traumatismes Presse Méd., 73:873-876, 1965.
18. Lucido, J. L., and Wall, C. A.: Rupture of diaphragm due to blunt trauma. Arch. Surg., 86:989-999, 1963.
19. Manlove, C. H., and Baranofsky, I. D.: Traumatic rupture of both leaves of the diaphragm. Surgery, 37:461-462, 1955.
20. Maurer, E. R.: Late sequelae of traumatic eventration of the diaphragm and their surgical management. Amer. Surgeon, 22:1194-1206, 1956.
21. Moreau, J.. La rupture du diaphragme doux les grandes contusions. J. Chir. (Paris), 74:46-71, 1957.
22. Neal, J. W.: Traumatic right diaphragmatic hernia with evisceration of stomach, transverse colon and liver into the right thorax. Ann. Surg., 137:281-284, 1953.
23. Nelson, J. B., Ziperman, H. H., Christensen, N. M., and Mathewson, C.: Diaphragmatic injuries and herniae. J. Trauma, 2:36-58, 1962.
24. Peck, W. A., Jr.: Diaphragmatic liver hernia following trauma. Amer. J. Roentgenol., 78:99-108, 1957.
25. Perry, T., Francis, W., and Lonergan, J.: Traumatic diaphragmatic hernia. Arch. Surg., 75:763-769, 1951.
26. Ramstrom, S., and Alesen, S.: Diaphragmatic rupture following abdominal injuries. Acta Chir. Scand., 107:304-308, 1954.
27. Schinz, H. R., et al: Roentgen Diagnosis. Vol. 3, Thorax. New York, Grune & Stratton, 1953.
28. Schneider, C. F.: Traumatic diaphragmatic hernia. Amer. J. Surg., 90:987-993, 1955.

12

LACERATION OF THE KIDNEY AND URETER

CLINICAL OBSERVATIONS

The organ most commonly injured in abdominal trauma is the kidney.[38] This high frequency is more apparent than real since very slight contusion of the kidney causes blood in the urine, whereas injury to other intra-abdominal organs is not so readily detectable.

Renal injury is suspect when there is pain and tenderness in the kidney regions with gross or microscopic blood in the urine. The patient may show contusion of the soft tissues over the flanks.

In addition to a direct blow to the abdomen, the kidney may be injured by the whiplash effect of a fall. The downward motion of the kidney continues, pulling on the pedicle. Some injuries have been attributed solely to vigorous muscle action on the part of the patient.[34]

An anomalous kidney, a hypertrophied kidney, or one involved by tumor or infection is more susceptible to injury. This possibility arises when hematuria follows a trivial blow (Fig. 12.1).[6, 29]

ASSOCIATED INJURIES

Fracture of the lower ribs posteriorly or of the transverse processes of the lumbar spine sometimes accompanies kidney injury. On the right side, kidney injury is associated with laceration of the liver, and on the left, with laceration of the spleen.

RADIOGRAPHIC EXAMINATION

Plain Film

The initial plain film of the abdomen shows the size, shape and position of the kidneys and whether the psoas muscles are symmetrical or obliterated by extravasated urine and hemorrhage.

A normal variation in the visualization of the psoas outlines has been shown by Elkin and Cohen.[9] They reviewed the abdominal films on 200 asymptomatic patients. Visualization was unequal in 25 per cent on single study and 11 per cent on multiple study. Absence of one psoas was found in 7.5 per cent on single study and 2.5 per cent on multiple study.

With this degree of variation in an asymptomatic population, impaired visualization of one psoas outline on a single film is of limited diagnostic value. If, however, unilateral loss of the psoas outline is accompanied by loss of the renal outline, and if there is inferior and medial displacement of the overlying colon, a retroperitoneal hemorrhage is likely. Continued bleeding into the retroperitoneal tissues is taking place when serial films show progressive obscuration of the psoas outline.

The spine is usually tilted to the injured side because of concomitant contusion of the ipsilateral lumbar and psoas muscles.

Intravenous Urography

An early urogram is recommended for every patient with suspected renal injury, not only to assess the degree of renal impairment, but to determine that the uninjured kidney is normal and functioning well. If the patient has a traumatic rupture of a congenital solitary kidney, this must be known prior to surgery.[1, 21, 43] Even without bowel preparation or dehydration, the urogram will give this information unless the patient is severely hypotensive.[8] Liska[17] recommends delayed films (at 2, 4 or 6 hours) when the traumatized kidney is not immediately visualized. In non-operative treatment of renal injuries, the course of healing is best assessed by serial urograms.[23]

Retrograde Pyelography

The need for retrograde pyelography is controversial. It is difficult to accomplish in the patient in shock, and carries with it the risk of introducing infection to the damaged kidney or of initiating further bleeding.[36, 42] In the author's experience, the technical quality of films obtained on intravenous urography is superior to those obtained on retrograde study. Little additional diagnostic information is obtained from the retrograde pyelogram. A contrary opinion is expressed by Orkin,[26, 27] who found retrograde study with cystoscopy to be more valuable than excretion urog-

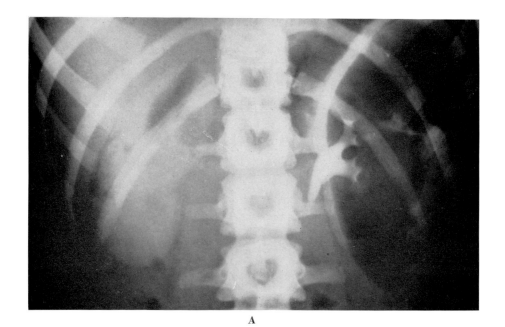

A

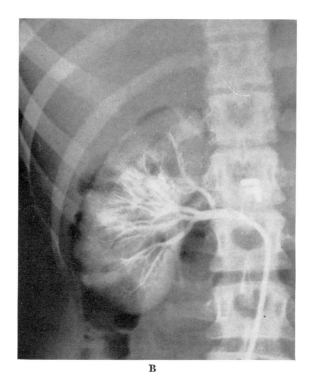

B

Figure 12.1.   *Continued on opposite page.*

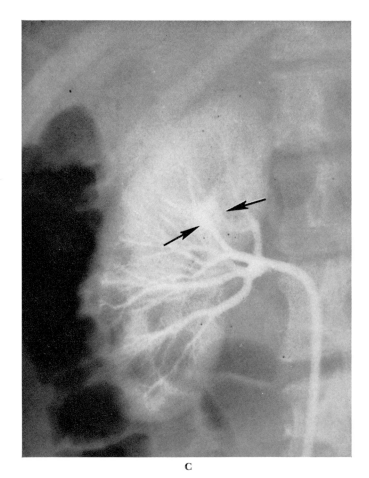

C

**FIGURE 12.1. BLEEDING INDUCED BY MINOR TRAUMA;
ARTERIOVENOUS MALFORMATION OF THE KIDNEY.**

A, Intravenous urogram. W.S., after a trivial blow to the abdomen, entered with
pain on the right side and bloody urine. No excretion on the right was seen.
Two days later, function of the right kidney had returned. *B,* Right renal
arteriogram, anteroposterior, third day. Adjacent to the hilum there is a cluster
of dilated tortuous small arterioles. *C,* Right renal arteriogram, right posterior
oblique. These vessels communicate with dilated veins which fill more rapidly
than the veins of the remainder of the kidney (arrows).

raphy and recommends that it be done routinely in every case of renal injury. Retrograde pyelography can be within normal limits in the presence of severe injury to the vascular pedicle.[46]

Intravenous Infusion Urography

An intravenous infusion urogram is useful in studying injured kidneys. Two milliliters of 25 per cent diatrizoate sodium per pound of body weight is infused intravenously and rapidly through a No. 18 needle.[33] A dense nephrogram is produced in about 10 minutes after the start of the infusion. Standard films and tomograms are taken.

Renal Scan

Radioactive isotope scanning of the kidneys is used when no excretion occurs on intravenous urography or when the patient has an allergy to iodides. An area of low uptake on the scan reflects vascular damage to that portion of the kidney (Fig. 12.19).

Renal Arteriography

The radiologist can best evaluate renal vascular injury by arteriography. It is most valuable in the study of a nonfunctioning kidney or when the pelvis is obstructed by blood clots. It can be done by retrograde femoral or axillary artery catheterization, or by retrograde brachial injection. Copek and Fojtik[4] report that arteriography is useful in children, and they have shown areas of ischemia of the renal tissue with displacement of ruptured segments. By defining the extent of vascular damage, a renal arteriogram helps the surgeon to decide whether operation or conservative therapy is indicated.[3, 10] Post-traumatic renal artery thrombosis can be demonstrated by arteriography.[14]

Kittredge et al.[15] studied the arteriographic changes taking place in the kidneys of dogs following induced trauma. In the minimal lesion group, no change was seen in the arterial pattern. In the nephrogram phase (capillary) a haziness of the cleft defect occurred. Prone and supine examination is recommended. Olsson and Lunderquist,[24] in 13 cases, found that arteriography determines when and where reparative surgery is needed.

TYPES OF INJURY

Glenn and Harvard[12] have a useful classification based on the radiographic manifestations and reflecting the severity of damage:

1. Simple contusion with no radiographic changes.

2. Minimal injury: intrarenal fracture beneath an intact capsule.
3. Moderate injury: laceration of the kidney with intrarenal or peri-renal hemorrhage.
4. Severe injury: fragmentation of the kidney or tear of the vascular pedicle.

Simple Contusion with No Radiographic Changes

Simple bruising with ecchymoses is the most common renal injury. It causes pain in the renal area and microscopic hematuria. The intravenous urogram is normal and the outlines of the kidney and psoas muscles are intact. After a few days of conservative treatment, pain subsides and hematuria disappears.

Minimal Injury: Intrarenal Fracture Beneath an Intact Capsule

Minimal injury due to intrarenal fracture leads to delayed excretion and decreased concentration (Fig. 12.2) because of edema and congestion

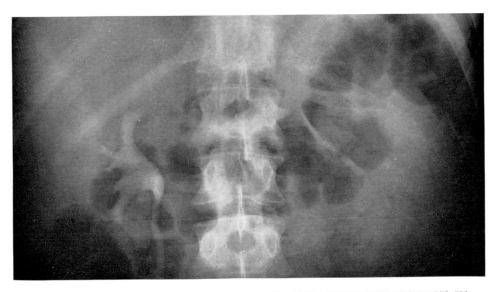

FIGURE 12.2. MINIMAL INJURY TO THE KIDNEY; SLIGHT DIMINUTION IN EXCRETION ON THE INVOLVED SIDE.

J.R. was seen with hematuria and pain in the left back after a fall. Both kidneys are of normal size and the psoas muscles are symmetrical. Excretion is slightly impaired on the left in comparison with the right kidney. Within two days the blood had disappeared from the urine and the patient had no further symptoms.

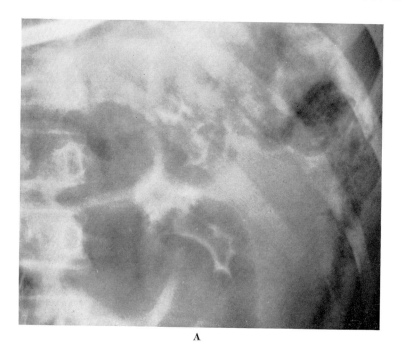

A

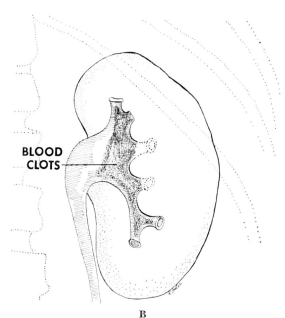

BLOOD
CLOTS

B

**FIGURE 12.3. MINIMAL INJURY TO THE KIDNEY;
INTRACALYCEAL AND INTRAPELVIC BLOOD CLOTS.**

A, Intravenous urogram. I. L. had been struck by an automobile and had bloody urine and pain in the left abdomen. Multiple fractures of the left lower ribs were noted. Diminished excretion is seen on the left side. *B,* Diagram. Blood clots cause filling defects within the calyces and pelvis. The outline of the left kidney is not seen.

of the kidney parenchyma as well as a reflex vasospasm so that blood is shunted away from injured glomeruli.[5] With gross bleeding, clots form a cast of the collecting structures (Fig. 12.3). Direct injury distorts the calyces and pelvis (Figs. 12.4 and 12.5). The outline of the kidney and psoas muscle remains intact.

Moderate Injury: Laceration of the Kidney with Intrarenal or Perirenal Hemorrhage

Moderate injury to the kidney is shown by enlargement of the renal outline or extravasation of the contrast medium on intravenous urography. Enlargement of the kidney results from edema and hemorrhage into the parenchyma or hemorrhage beneath the capsule of the kidney.[13] With bleeding limited to the kidney, the sharp renal outline is intact (Fig. 12.6). With perirenal hemorrhage, the kidney outline is lost because the perirenal fat is infiltrated by extravasated blood (Fig. 12.7). The perirenal fat is also separated from the kidney.

Extravasation of opaque medium is found when the damage is limited to one pole. The unaffected portion of the kidney continues to excrete and the opaque medium leaks from the torn calyx or pelvis (Fig. 12.8). It is a relatively infrequent finding in renal injury.

Severe Injury: Fragmentation of the Kidney or Tear of the Vascular Pedicle

Severe injury causes an extensive leak of blood and urine into the retroperitoneal space. This type is less common and generally requires surgical treatment. Hemorrhage completely obscures the kidney and psoas muscles (Figs. 12.9 and 12.10). As the blood surrounds the kidney within Gerota's fascia, it displaces the perirenal fat peripherally. A large mass, consisting of renal fragments and hematoma, is outlined by fat. There is often a scoliosis of the lumbar spine, concave toward the involved side. The large hematoma surrounding the lacerated kidney displaces the colon medially and inferiorly (Figs. 3.20, 12.12, 12.13).

An apparent density is found between the displaced colon and the lateral properitoneal fat line. This simulates intraperitoneal blood (Figs. 12.12 and 12.13). It is differentiated from intraperitoneal bleeding by the fact that the kidney and psoas are obscured. Furthermore, there is no blood in the opposite flank or pelvis.

Excretion of the urographic medium is usually absent, but if present, there is deformity of the calyces and pelvis. The hemorrhagic mass displaces the ureter and bladder medially (Fig. 12.11).

As long as hemorrhage is limited and infection is absent, most kidney injuries are treated conservatively.[20, 22] This requires continued clinical

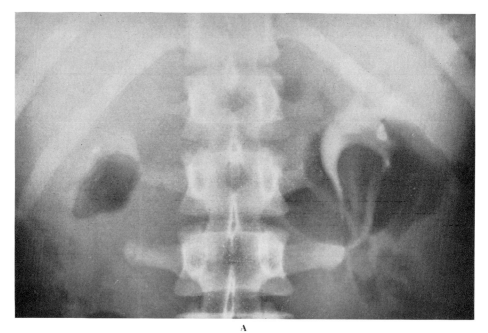

A

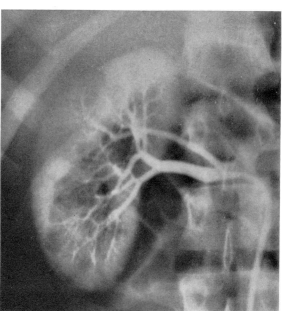

B

**FIGURE 12.4. MINIMAL INJURY OF THE RIGHT KIDNEY WITH DIMINISHED
EXCRETION AND CALYCEAL IRREGULARITY.**

A, Intravenous urogram. R.M. sustained a blow to the right flank and six hours
later had gross hematuria. The urogram shows impaired excretion on the right
side with irregularity of the middle and inferior calyces. *B,* Selective right renal
arteriogram. Four days later, the arteriogram is within normal limits and there
is no evidence of endarteritis or extravasation (the peripheral radiolucency is
due to technique). Intravenous urography after one month showed normal
appearance of the injured calyces.

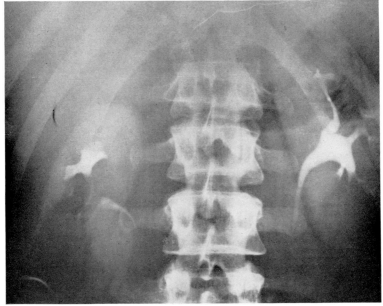

A

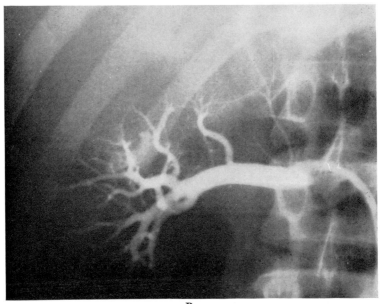

B

FIGURE 12.5. MINIMAL INJURY OF THE RIGHT KIDNEY; IRREGULARITY OF THE MIDDLE AND INFERIOR CALYCES; FOLLOW-UP SELECTIVE RENAL ARTERIOGRAPHY SHOWING A NORMAL VASCULAR TREE.

A, Intravenous urogram. S. McN. had been beaten by a burglar. He had extreme tenderness over the right flank with microscopic hematuria. The right middle and inferior calyces are irregular. Right kidney outline and psoas muscle are intact. *B,* Renal arteriogram. A selective right renal arteriogram two weeks later shows a normal right renal artery with its branches. Hematuria subsided and the patient had no further symptoms.

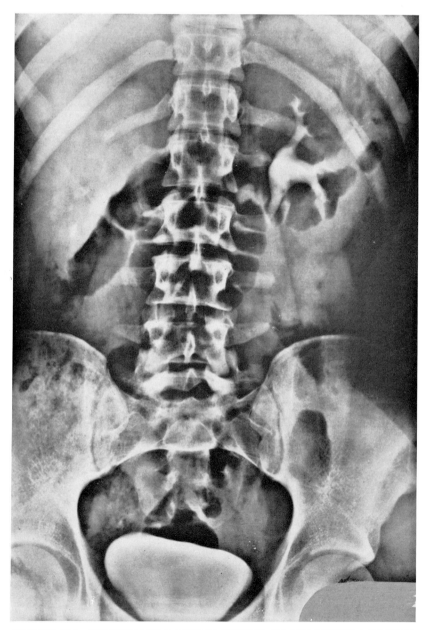

**FIGURE 12.6. MODERATELY SEVERE INJURY TO THE RIGHT KIDNEY;
ENLARGEMENT OF THE KIDNEY; IMPAIRED FUNCTION;
BLOOD CLOT FILLING THE BLADDER.**

K.M. had been kicked in a soccer game and had gross hematuria. On intravenous urography, excretion is diminished on the right and the right kidney is larger than the left both in length and transverse diameter. The sharp outline of the kidney is maintained, indicating that this is intrarenal hemorrhage and edema and not perirenal bleeding. A large blood clot fills the bladder.

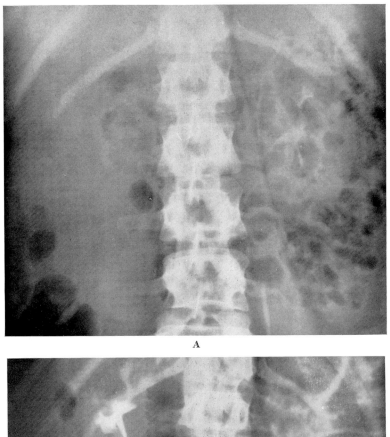

A

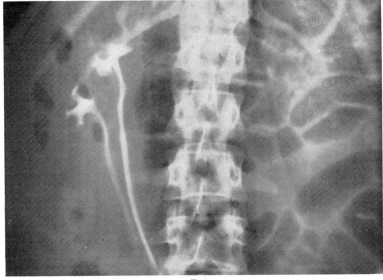

B

FIGURE 12.7. MODERATELY SEVERE INJURY TO THE KIDNEY SHOWN BY FAILURE TO EXCRETE THE CONTRAST MEDIUM AND BY COMPLETE OBSCURATION OF THE KIDNEY AND PSOAS OUTLINE.

A, Intravenous urogram. J.G., after an automobile accident, had right costovertebral angle tenderness and hematuria. There is complete obscuration of the right kidney shadow. No excretion of the contrast medium occurred on the right side up to 2 hours. (Reflex vasospasm?) *B,* Retrograde pyelogram. The following day, pyelography reveals normal calyces, bifid pelves and ureters. She was treated conservatively.

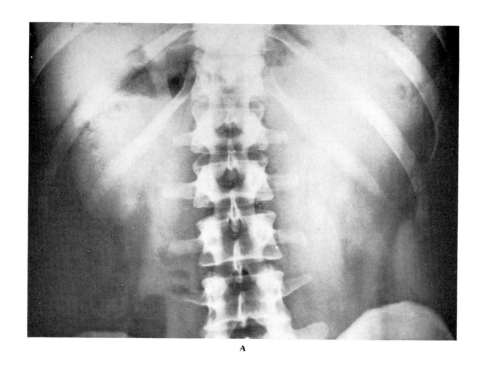

A

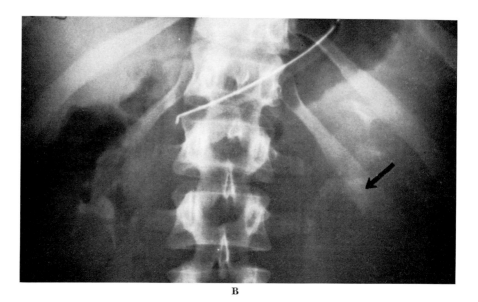

B

Figure 12.8. *Continued on opposite page.*

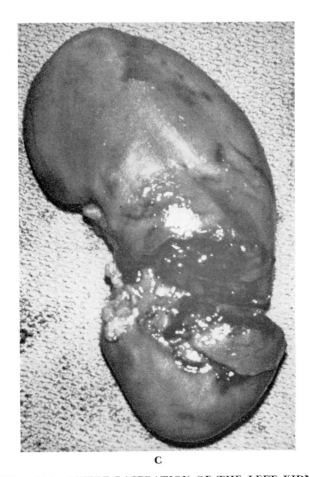

C

FIGURE 12.8. SEVERE LACERATION OF THE LEFT KIDNEY.

A, Plain film. J.D. In a motorcycle accident, the handle bar had jabbed him in the left abdomen. He had gross hematuria and the hematocrit was 32. The lower half of the left kidney is obscured in comparison with the right. There is also obscuration of the upper margin of the left psoas. The lumbar spine is con cave to the left. *B,* Five minute intravenous urogram. There is impaired excre tion on the left side. Intraparenchymal extravasation is seen about the inferior calyx (arrow). *C,* Photograph of specimen. Because of a continued fall in the hematocrit, left nephrectomy was done. A large amount of blood sur rounded the torn kidney.

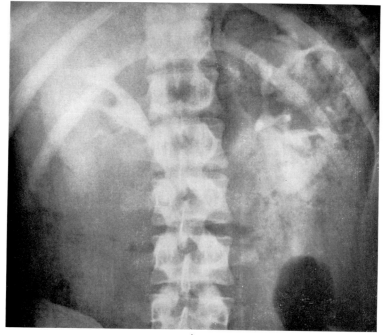

A

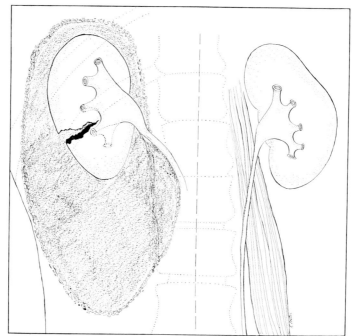

B

FIGURE 12.9. SEVERE INJURY TO THE KIDNEY; RETROPERITONEAL HEMATOMA.

A, Intravenous urogram. R.A. had right upper quadrant pain with hematuria. There is loss of the right psoas outlines with a tilt of the spine to the right side. A perirenal mass is seen and the right inferior calyx is irregular. *B,* Diagram. At operation, a mass of clotted blood surrounded the kidney from a laceration on the posterior surface.

observation and repeated urographic study. Renal surgery is preferably performed after the patient's clinical condition has stabilized. With small perirenal hematomas, absorption takes place; calcification of the hematoma is rarely seen.[31]

COMPLICATIONS OF RENAL INJURY

Perinephric Abscess

Perinephric abscess may complicate renal injury with extravasation and will appear in about two to six weeks (Figs. 12.14 and 12.15). When adherent to the kidney, it will distort the calyces and renal vessels and obscure the renal outline. The abscess may point into the flank or into the groin. Incision and drainage are required.[19]

Delayed Renal Hemorrhage

This may occur after an interval of many weeks (Fig. 12.16). The radiographic findings depend on the severity of the blood loss and whether it takes place into the perirenal tissues or into the collecting system. To reduce this possibility, patients with kidney injury are placed on bed rest until they are asymptomatic and the urine is clear.[34]

Renal Atrophy

When a portion of the kidney loses its blood supply, atrophy with deformity of the calyceal structures results (Fig. 12.17).[16] Whether this causes subsequent hypertension is conjectural. Cases have been reported in which hypertension followed trauma to the kidney and was relieved by nephrectomy.[11, 47] In a follow-up study of two children with atrophy of the kidney following trauma, Palavatona, Graham and Silverman[28] found no associated clinical manifestations. Slade, Evans and Roylance[36] followed up 59 patients with closed renal injury. Only when calyceal rupture occurred did an alteration in kidney architecture result. Nearly all these patients had good renal function and all were symptom-free and normotensive. Opit et al.[25] found good renal function as assessed by pyelography in a follow-up of 77 patients with closed renal injury.

INJURY TO THE URETER

Tear of the ureter is a rare occurrence following blunt trauma to the abdomen; only a few cases have been reported. It may be manifested only by hematuria, often microscopic.[39] In most reported cases, the ureter has been injured at the ureteropelvic juncture (Fig. 12.18).

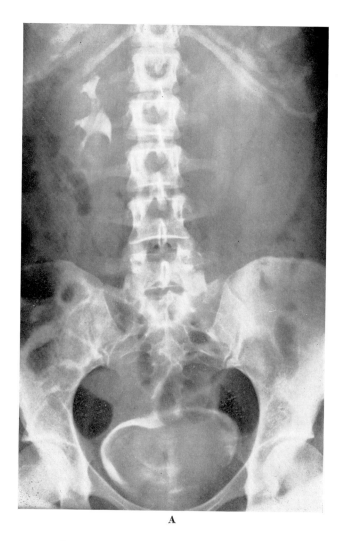

A

Figure 12.10. *Continued on opposite page.*

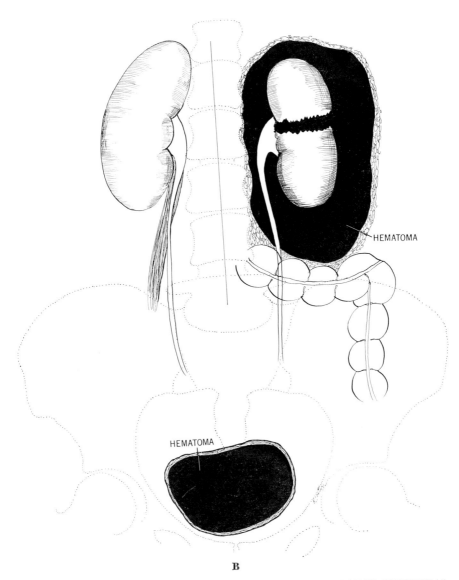

HEMATOMA

HEMATOMA

B

**FIGURE 12.10. SEVERE INJURY TO THE LEFT KIDNEY; LARGE PERIRENAL
HEMATOMA; BLOOD CLOT IN BLADDER.**

A, Intravenous urogram. N.C. had urgency, bloody urine and left flank tenderness. The left kidney is surrounded by a hematoma which has displaced the colon
inferiorly and obscured the psoas muscle. There is a left concavity of the
lumbar spine. No opaque medium was excreted from the left kidney. A blood
clot forms a cast of the bladder. *B,* Diagram. At operation, the kidney was
found to be fragmented, with massive retroperitoneal hematoma surrounding
the kidney fragments.

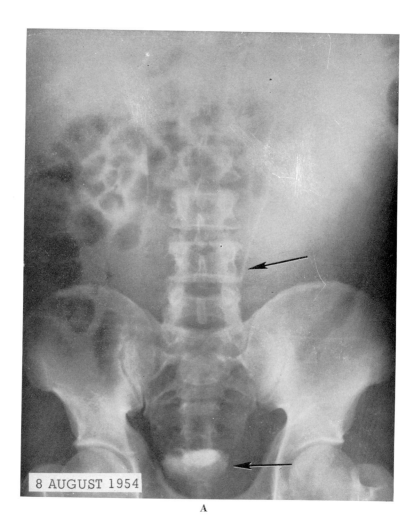

8 AUGUST 1954

A

Figure 12.11. *Continued on opposite page.*

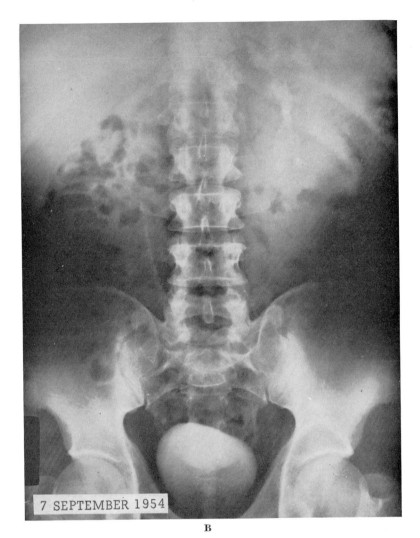

7 SEPTEMBER 1954

B

**FIGURE 12.11. SEVERE INJURY OF THE LEFT KIDNEY; RETROPERITONEAL
HEMATOMA DISPLACING THE URETER AND BLADDER.**

A, Initial intravenous urogram. A.R., after an alcoholic spree, had pain in the
left abdomen. The urine was grossly bloody. Only the superior calyces on the
left side are visualized. The left kidney and psoas muscle are obscured by perinephric hematoma, which displaces the left ureter (upper arrow) and bladder
(lower arrow) to the right. *B,* Intravenous urogram one month later. The
perirenal hematoma has been almost completely absorbed. Displacement of
the ureter and bladder is no longer present.

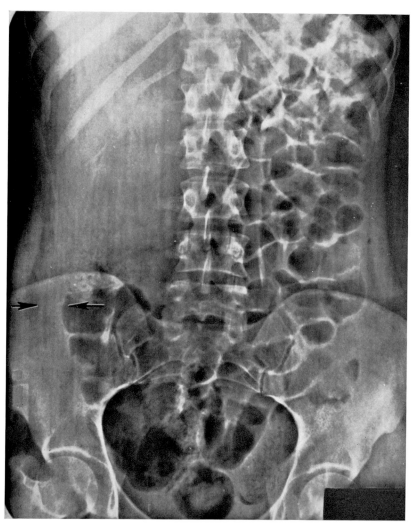

FIGURE 12.12. SEVERE INJURY TO THE KIDNEY; RETROPERITONEAL HEMATOMA DISPLACING THE LARGE AND SMALL BOWEL INFERIORLY AND MEDIALLY.

J.M. had been thrown from a car and had tenderness in the right upper abdomen. A large retroperitoneal hematoma obscures the right kidney and displaces the gas-filled intestines inferiorly and medially. It extends retroperitoneally between the ascending colon and the properitoneal fat (arrows). No excretion occurs on the right. The hematoma within Gerota's fascia was due to complete rupture of the right kidney.

(Illustration on opposite page.)

FIGURE 12.13. SEVERE INJURY TO THE RIGHT KIDNEY; KIDNEY FRAGMENTS SURROUNDED BY LARGE PERIRENAL HEMATOMA; NEPHROGRAPHIC EFFECT ON UROGRAPHY.

A, Intravenous urogram. J.L. had fallen, striking the right flank. A large mass obscures the kidney and psoas muscle on the right. The right kidney is dense (nephrographic effect) with a surrounding mass (perirenal hematoma). No opacification of the calyces, pelves or ureter occurred. *B,* Diagram. Note medial and inferior displacement of colon. At operation, the upper pole of the right kidney was found to be completely transected and surrounded by a large hematoma within Gerota's fascia.

194

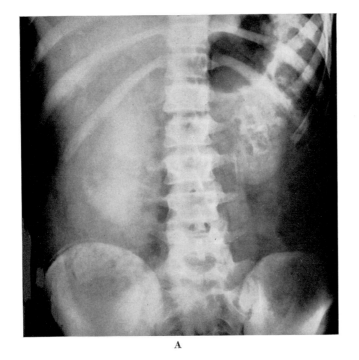

A

B

Figure 12.13.   *Legend on opposite page*

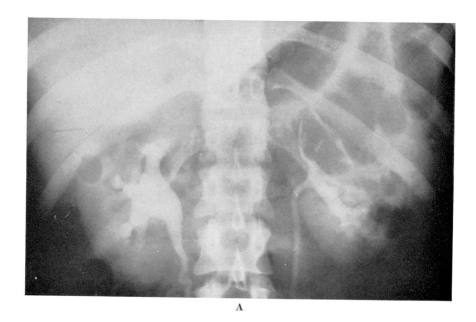

A

Figure 12.14. *Continued on opposite page.*

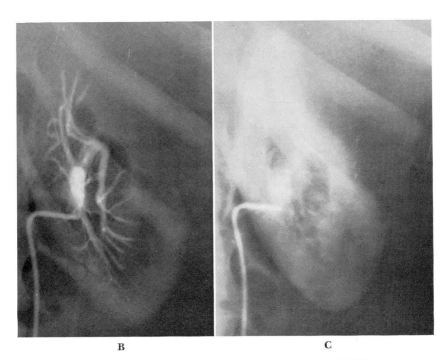

B   C

FIGURE 12.14. INFECTED PERINEPHRIC HEMATOMA.

A, Intravenous urogram. B.R. had been beaten and kicked in a fight 6 weeks before entry. He had left costovertebral angle pain and fever spikes to 104°. This film shows the calyces and pelvis of the left kidney that are compressed by a mass in the upper outer segment.   *B,* Selective arteriography, arterial phase. Both the dorsal and ventral branches of the renal artery are displaced. No arterial occlusion or abnormal vessels are seen.   *C,* Selective arteriography, capillary phase. The upper outer segment of the kidney does not opacify. On the following day, an infected perirenal hematoma was opened and drained.

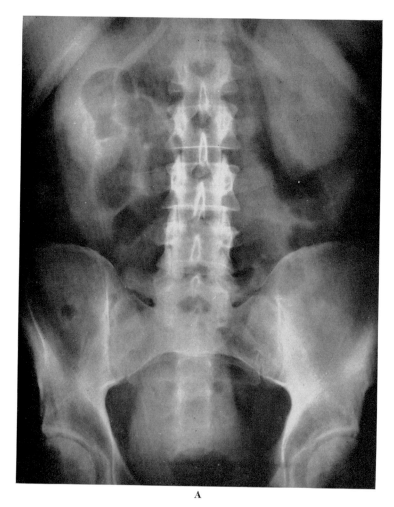

A

FIGURE 12.15. RETROPERITONEAL ABSCESS FOLLOWING LACERATION OF THE KIDNEY; ABSCESS CAVITY OUTLINED BY CONTRAST MEDIUM.

A, Intravenous urogram. For five days O.E. had had pain in the left groin. The left kidney is larger than the right, but smooth in outline. The bladder is displaced to the right. Exploratory laparotomy revealed a retroperitoneal abscess containing necrotic fat, blood and urine from a tear in the anterior surface of the kidney. *B*, Anteroposterior film after injection of diatrizoate sodium. The abscess cavity is anterior and lateral to the left kidney. *C*, Lateral film after injection. The abscess cavity extends into the left inguinal area.

(Continued on opposite page.)

(Illustration on opposite page.)

FIGURE 12.16. DELAYED RUPTURE OF THE KIDNEY (TWO MONTHS).

W.T., after a fall, was examined and no urinary tract abnormality was discovered. Two months later, he experienced a sudden onset of severe continuous left flank pain radiating into the left hip. On intravenous urogram, a large mass replaces the left kidney and obscures the left psoas muscle. There is no excretion on the left side. A large perirenal hematoma due to laceration of the lower pole of the left kidney was found.

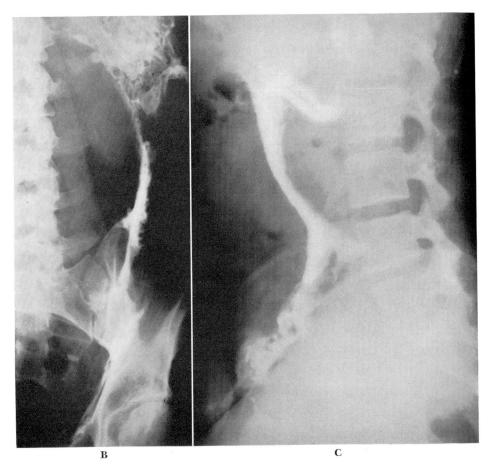

B   C

Figure 12.15. *Legend on opposite page.*

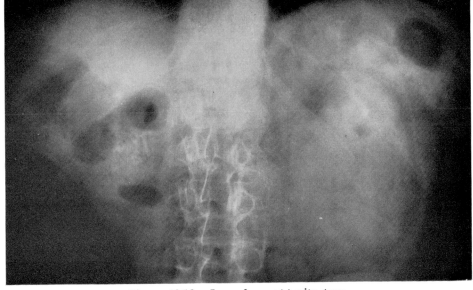

Figure 12.16. *Legend on opposite page.*

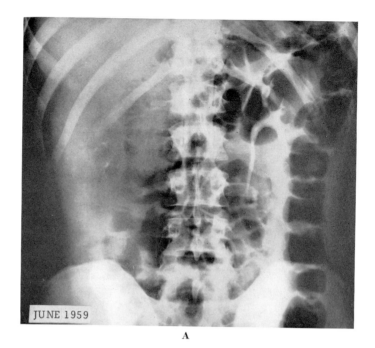

A

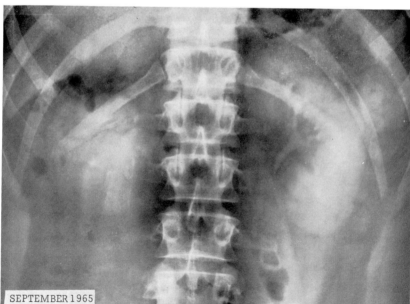

B

**FIGURE 12.17.   SEVERE INJURY TO RIGHT KIDNEY; POST-TRAUMATIC
RENAL ATROPHY; HYPERTENSION.**

A, Intravenous urogram. D.M. had injured the right kidney in an automobile
accident. Excretion is impaired and only the middle and inferior calyces on the
right are visualized. A large hematoma surrounds the kidney. It displaces the

(Continued on opposite page.)

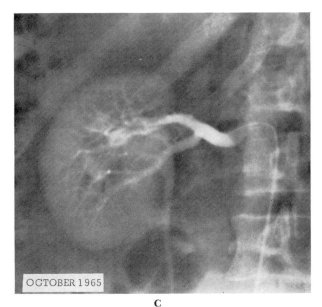

OCTOBER 1965

C

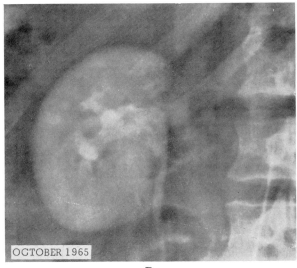

OCTOBER 1965

D

ascending colon inferiorly and medially and is seen in the retroperitoneal tissues between colon and properitoneal fat. Treatment was nonoperative and the hematuria cleared after two weeks of bed rest. *B,* Intravenous urogram, 6 years later. At the age of 24 years a blood pressure of 180/100 was found on a preemployment physical examination. The right kidney is 4.5 cm. shorter than the left, with contraction of the upper pole. *C,* Selective right arteriogram, arterial phase. No arterial narrowing or deformity is demonstrable. That the hypertension results from the renal injury is not proved. *D,* Selective right arteriogram, capillary phase. The upper half of the kidney is shrunken in comparison with the lower half.

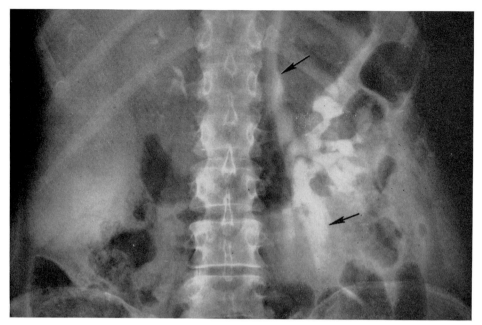

**FIGURE 12.18.   LACERATION OF URETER AT URETEROPELVIC JUNCTION;
EXTRAVASATION.**

E.B. had gross hematuria with left costovertebral angle tenderness and a fracture
to the left 12th rib posteriorly. There is extravasation of the contrast medium
from a tear in the pelvis above the ureteral pelvic junction. The medium extends
retroperitoneally along the psoas muscle (arrows). Blood clots are present within
the pelvis of the kidney.

Wilenius,[45] in an experimental study, found that in ureteral injuries
caused by wheels rolling across the abdomen, tears of the ureter are most
common at the level of the 2nd, 3rd and 5th lumbar vertebrae.

When there is no associated injury of the kidney or its vascular supply,
urine will continue to form. This urine leaks into the soft tissues at
the site of the injury, forming a large urinary cyst that is palpable either
in the flank or anteriorly.[2, 18, 30, 32, 35, 37]

Pararenal pseudocysts result from urinary extravasation and displace
the kidney upward, but a definite line of separation is seen between the
cyst and the kidney.[44, 48] If infection supervenes, there are tenderness, fever
and leukocytosis.[7] On intravenous urography, the kidney may excrete
normally, or a slight hydronephrosis may be present. In some instances,
the ureter is obstructed; in others, extravasation occurs from the open
end.[40] In the patient of Sturdy and Magell,[41] the cyst emptied completely
with a change in the patient's position. Drainage of the collection of
urine and reconstruction of the ureter are the recommended treatment.[35]

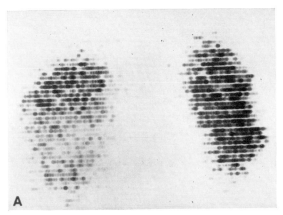
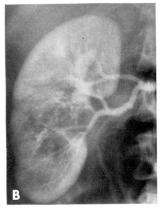

FIGURE 12.19. MODERATELY SEVERE INJURY OF KIDNEY.

R.C. had hematuria after injury. *A*, Renal scan. The lower right kidney is avascular. *B*, Selective right renal arteriogram. Arterial phase. In the avascular area, the vessels are distorted.

REFERENCES

1. Anderson, E. E., and Harrison, J. H.: Surgical importance of the solitary kidney. New Engl. J. Med., *273*:683-687, 1965.
2. Blancato, C.: Pseudoidonephrosi da rottura traumatica completa dell' uretre. Chirurgia, *12*:16-21, 1957.
3. Braedel, H. U.: Renal angiography after blunt trauma to the kidney. Fortschr. Roentgenstr., *99*:416-418, 1963.
4. Capek, V., and Fojtik, F.: The significance of selective renal angiography in injuries of the kidney in childhood. Amer. J. Roentgenol., *90*:75-82, 1963.
5. Chovnick, S. D., and Newman, H. R.: Management of renal injuries. J. Urol., *83*:330-336, 1960.
6. Cope, J. C.: Traumatic rupture of a congenital solitary kidney. J. Urol., *92*:377, 1964.
7. Crosby, D. L.: An unusual case of renal trauma. Brit. J. Urol., *31*:159-160, 1959.
8. Dowse, J. L. A., and Kihn, R. B.: Renal injuries. Diagnosis, management and sequelae in 67 cases. Brit. J. Surg., *50*:353-361, 1963.
9. Elkin, M., and Cohen, G.: Diagnostic value of psoas shadow. Clin. Radiol., *13*:210-217, 1962.
10. Frost, B.: Selektive renale Angiographie bei Nierenruptur. Beschreibung des Falles. Fortschr. Roentgenstrahl., *92*:260-262, 1962.
11. Gibson, G. R.: Ruptured horseshoe (fused) kidney: A review and report of a case with traumatic renal hypertension. J. Urol., *92*:374-376, 1964.
12. Glenn, J. F., and Harvard, B. M.: The injured kidney. J.A.M.A., *173*:1189-1195, 1960.
13. Gremmel, H.: Instant roentgenologic diagnosis in vascular trauma and vascular occlusion. Radiologe, *3*:455-461, 1963.
14. Henley, S. D., and Finby, N.: Renal trauma. A concept of injury to the renal artery. Radiology, *79*:816-821, 1962.
15. Kittredge, R. D., Iswariah, J., Draper, J., and Finby, N.: Experimental kidney laceration, rupture and amputation. Amer. J. Roentgenol., *93*:891-897, 1965.
16. Lagarde, C., Perruchio, P., and Raveleau, R.: Atrophie renale post traumatique: document radiologiques. J. Radiol. Electr., *39*:797-798, 1958.
17. Liska, J. R.: Recognition and management of trauma to the kidney. J. Urol., *78*:525-531, 1957.
18. Lloyd, F. A.: War injuries of ureter. Bull. Northwestern Univ. Med. School, *30*:74-79, 1956.

19. Lombardo, L. J., Heyman, A. M., and Barnes, R. W.: Injuries to the urinary tract due to external trauma. J.A.M.A., *172*:1618-1622, 1960.
20. Mayor, G.: Prinzipielle Fragen bei Nierenverletzungen. Urol. Int., *11*:368-385, 1961.
21. Murphy, J. J., Iozzi, L., and Schoenberg, H. W.: Principles of management of renal trauma. J. Trauma, *2*:327-336, 1962.
22. Nation, E. F., and Massey, B. D.: Management of renal trauma. J. Urol., *89*: 775-778, 1963.
23. Nillson, J., and Sandberg, N.: Healing of kidney injuries: Clinical and roentgenographic follow-up study. Acta Chir. Scand., *123*:228-240, 1962.
24. Olsson, O., and Lunderquist, A.: Angiography in renal trauma. Acta Radiol., *1*:1-20, 1963.
25. Opit, L. J., McKenna, K. P., and Nairn, D. E.: Closed renal injury. Brit. J. Surg., *48*:240-247, 1960.
26. Orkin, L. A.: Evaluation of the merits of cystoscopy and retrograde pyelography in the management of renal trauma. J. Urol.,*63*:9-24, 1950.
27. Orkin, L. A.: The diagnosis of urological trauma in presence of other injuries. Surg. Clin. North America, *33*:1473-1496, 1953.
28. Palavatana, C., Graham, S. R., and Silverman, F. N.: Delayed sequels to renal injury in childhood. Amer. J. Roentgenol., *91*:659-665, 1964.
29. Persky, L., and Forsythe, W. E.: Renal trauma in childhood. J.A.M.A., *182*: 709-712, 1962.
30. Pyrah, L. N., and Smiddy, F. G.: Pararenal pseudohydronephrosis. A report of two cases. Brit. J. Urol., *25*:239-246, 1953.
31. Salik, J. O., and Abeshouse, B. S.: Calcification, ossification and cartilage formation in the kidney. Amer. J. Roentgenol., *88*:125-143, 1962.
32. Sauls, C. L., and Nesbit, P. M.: Pararenal pseudocysts: A report of four cases. J. Urol., *87*:288-296, 1962.
33. Schencker, B., Marcure, R. W., and Moody, D. L.: Simplified nephrotomography; the dry infusion technique. Amer. J. Roentgenol., *95*:283-290, 1965.
34. School, A. J., and Nation, E. F.: Chapter 18, Injuries of the kidney. *In* Campbell, M. F. (ed.): Urology. 2nd ed. Philadelphia, W. B. Saunders Co., 1963.
35. Seright, W.: Traumatic closed rupture of upper ureter. Brit. J. Surg., *46*:511-514, 1958-1959.
36. Slade, N., Evans, K. T., and Roylance, J.: Late results of closed renal injuries. Brit. J. Surg., *49*:194-196, 1962.
37. Smith, M. J. V., Nanson, E. M., and Campbell, J. M.: An unusual case of closed rupture of the ureter. J. Urol., *83*:277-278, 1960.
38. Solheim, K.: Closed abdominal injuries. Acta Chir. Scand., *126*:574-592, 1963.
39. Stickel, D. L., and Howse, R. M.: Injuries of the ureter due to external violence. Review of literature and report of 2 cases. Ann. Surg., *154*:137-141, 1961.
40. Stone, H. H., and Jones, H. Q.: Penetrating and nonpenetrating injuries to the ureter. Surg. Gynec. Obstet., *114*:52-68, 1962.
41. Sturdy, D. E., and Magell, J.: Traumatic perinephric cyst (pseudohydronephrosis). Brit. J. Surg., *48*:315-318, 1961.
42. True, E.: De la nécessité des explorations uroradiologiques dans les traumatismes des reins. Mem. Acad. Chir., *77*:594-596, 1951.
43. Turton, J. R. H., and Williamson, J. Traumatic rupture of congenital solitary kidney. Brit. J. Surg., *23*:327-337, 1935.
44. Weintraub, H. O., Rall, K. L., Thompson, I. M., and Ross, G.: Pararenal pseudocysts. Amer. J. Roentgenol., *92*:286-290, 1964.
45. Wilenius, R.: Subcutaneous rupture of the ureter. Ann. Chir. et Gynaec. Fenniae, *39*:1, 1950.
46. Willi-Baumkauff, H.: Zur Rontgenuntersuchung bei Nierenverletzungen. Monatsschr. Unfallh. *53*:289-301, 1950.
47. Zimmerman, S. J., and Radding, R. S.: Hypertension due to trauma of the kidney. New Engl. J. Med., *264*:238-240, 1961.
48. Zufall, R.: Traumatic avulsion of upper ureter. J. Urol., *85*:246-248, 1961.

13

LACERATION OF THE BLADDER

CLINICAL OBSERVATIONS

Bladder injury is suggested by retropubic pain, hematuria and extreme urgency.[6] The patient can void only small amounts of urine with difficulty, or cannot void at all.

ASSOCIATED INJURIES

Injuries to the bladder often accompany fractures of the pelvis located below the pelvic brim. Of 14 patients with bladder rupture seen at the Santa Clara County Hospital, 10 had pelvic fractures. Of 125 patients with pelvic fractures reported by Richardson,[9] 8 per cent had injuries to the bladder or urethra. Of 200 patients with pelvic fractures, Todd[10] found 4.6 per cent to have injuries to the bladder and urethra, and 10.8 per cent to have hematuria. Newland[7] suggests that every patient with a pelvic fracture should be investigated for possible damage to the lower urinary tract.

RADIOGRAPHIC EXAMINATION

Plain Film of Abdomen

Because the bladder is surrounded by perivesical fat, it can often be identified without the use of a contrast medium. The film of the abdomen is examined for pelvic fracture. If a fracture is present, a careful search is made for detached spicules of bone projecting into the bladder.[3] With intraperitoneal rupture, fluid will be found in the flanks or pelvis. Pneumoperitoneum has been reported when the patient with intraperitoneal rupture is catheterized prior to radiographic examination.[4] Retroperitoneal hematoma in the lateral pelvic wall displaces and compresses the bladder (Chapter 15).

Intravenous Urogram

The intravenous urogram is done to rule out concomitant injuries of the kidneys and ureters. When the kidneys and ureters are excluded as the cause of hematuria, attention is focused on the bladder. Bladder injury may be overlooked on the cystogram produced by excretory urography[11] because of either insufficient density of the contrast medium or pressure inadequate to produce leakage.

Retrograde Cystography

A retrograde cystogram is the single most important diagnostic study in bladder injury.[1] Under sterile conditions, a Foley balloon catheter is placed in the bladder and from 150 to 200 milliliters of water-soluble sterile iodide solution are run in by gravity. Films are taken in the anteroposterior, lateral and oblique projections. If the associated pelvic fractures contraindicate movement of the patient, the oblique films of the bladder are taken by angling the tube.

TYPES OF BLADDER LACERATION

Radiographically, three types of injury to the bladder have been encountered: (1) mucosal tear and contusion, (2) intraperitoneal rupture, and (3) retroperitoneal rupture. These may present individually or in combination. The most common bladder injury is contusion. Retroperitoneal bladder rupture is about four times more frequent than intraperitoneal.[6, 8]

Mucosal Tear and Contusion

A break in the mucosa is shown by a small intramural extravasation of the contrast medium (Fig. 13.1). Deformity and irregularity of the bladder wall due to spasm and edema are sometimes seen. Mucosal tears usually do not require surgical treatment. The majority of mucosal tears and contusions are undetectable radiographically, and are manifest only by transient hematuria following injury. The diagnosis is made by exclusion.

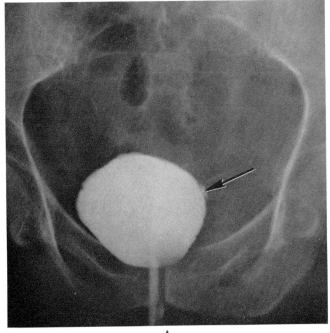

A

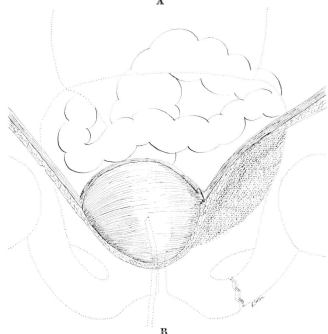

B

FIGURE 13.1. MUCOSAL TEAR AND CONTUSION OF THE BLADDER.

A, Cystogram. R.H. had a fracture of the left pubic bone with hematuria. The bladder is displaced toward the right by a pelvic hematoma adjacent to the pubic fractures. There is a collar-button-like projection on the left side of the urinary bladder (arrow). *B,* Diagram. The patient died shortly after admission and autopsy showed a rent in the mucosa on the left side of the urinary bladder, with hemorrhage into the muscularis.

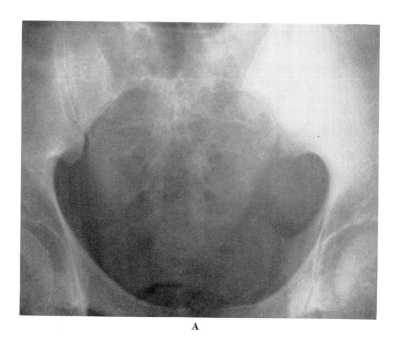

A

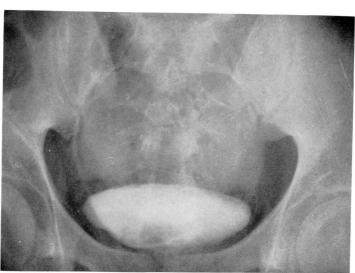

B

Figure 13.2. *Continued on opposite page.*

Intraperitoneal Rupture

Intraperitoneal rupture is more likely to follow a blow to the lower abdomen when the bladder is distended.[8] If a large amount of urine mixed with blood leaks into the peritoneal sac, it is seen in the flanks and pelvis on the plain film (Fig. 12.2*A*). After intravenous urography, the contrast medium is excreted by the kidneys, passes into the torn bladder and escapes into the peritoneal cavity. An increase in density of the intraperitoneal fluid after urography is diagnostic of intraperitoneal rupture (Fig. 13.2*B*).

Following retrograde cystography, the injected medium enters directly into the peritoneal cavity (Fig. 13.3). The loops of small and large bowel within the abdomen indent the contrast medium and produce scalloped

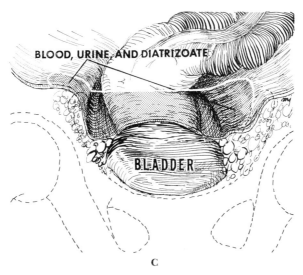

C

FIGURE 13.2. INTRAPERITONEAL RUPTURE OF THE BLADDER; INCREASED DENSITY OF PERITONEAL FLUID AFTER UROGRAPHY

A, Preliminary film. R.W. had grossly bloody urine after an automobile accident. Fluid is present in the pelvic recesses of the peritoneal cavity. *B,* Intravenous urogram. The fluid became increasingly dense after the urogram, indicating a leak of the opaque medium from the bladder. *C,* Diagram. At operation, there was a 10 cm. intraperitoneal rupture of the bladder dome, with approximately 800 milliliters of bloody urine in the peritoneal cavity.

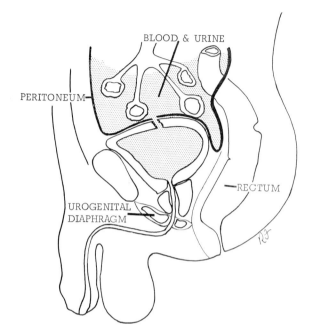

BLOOD & URINE

PERITONEUM

UROGENITAL
DIAPHRAGM

RECTUM

**FIGURE 13.3. DIAGRAM. INTRA-
PERITONEAL RUPTURE OF
BLADDER.**

Opaque medium, urine and
blood directly enter the peritoneal cavity. The gas-filled
loop of small bowel indents
the opaque fluid, producing
"scalloped defects."

defects, a reliable sign of intraperitoneal leakage from a torn bladder
(Figs. 13.4, 13.5 and 13.6).[2] A unique complication of intraperitoneal
rupture is herniation of a loop of small bowel into the bladder through
the defect in its wall (Fig. 13.7).

Retroperitoneal Rupture

When the base of the bladder is injured, urine and blood collect in
the retroperitoneal tissues and compress the bladder (Fig. 13.8). The diagnosis of retroperitoneal tear is made when the injected contrast material
extends streak-like into the retroperitoneal tissues and produces the
"sunburst" effect described by Weens[11] (Figs. 13.9, 13.10 and 13.11). The
outer wall of the bowel is not outlined as in intraperitoneal rupture. Urine
and blood in the retroperitoneal tissues elevate the bladder above the
pelvic floor (Figs. 13.12 and 13.13). Kaiser and Farrow[5] found that most
retroperitoneal tears occur on the anterolateral surface near the bladder neck.

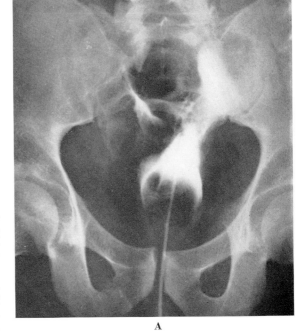

A

**FIGURE 13.4. INTRAPERITO-
NEAL RUPTURE OF THE
BLADDER; OPAQUE MEDIUM
COATING THE OUTER WALL
OF THE SIGMOID.**

A, Cystogram. C.C. had
multiple severe fractures of
the pelvis. The contrast medium passes into the peritoneal cavity, outlining the
outer wall of the sigmoid. *B,*
Diagram. A stellate laceration of the posterior-superior
margin of the bladder was
found.

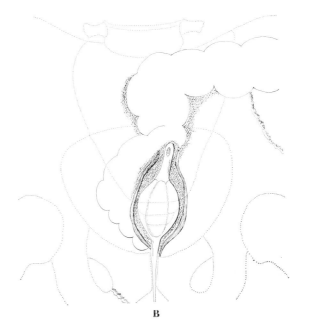

B

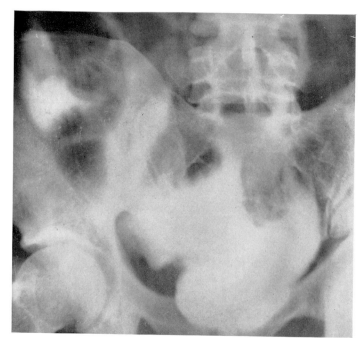

FIGURE 13.5.   INTRAPERITONEAL RUPTURE OF THE BLADDER.

R.A. had been in an automobile accident. Cystography shows the opaque medium entering the peritoneal cavity. The indentation of the opaque contrast
material by the dilated loops of bowel produces a typical scalloped appearance.

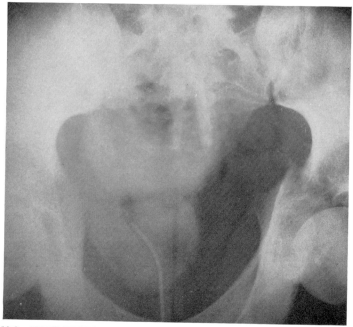

FIGURE 13.6.   INTRAPERITONEAL RUPTURE OF THE BLADDER; CYSTOGRAM.

T.S. had a posterior dislocation of the left hip. The opaque medium leaks into
the peritoneal cavity and surrounds the loops of bowel, producing a scalloped
effect. A large retroperitoneal hematoma about the fracture of the left acetabulum
displaces the bladder to the right.

212

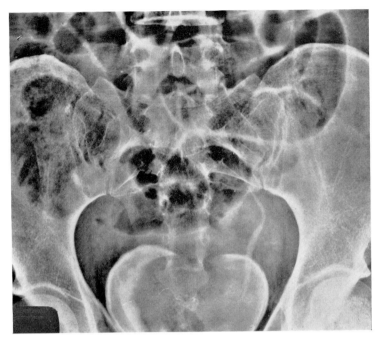

**FIGURE 13.7. INTRAPERITONEAL RUPTURE OF BLADDER;
SMALL BOWEL HERNIATION.**

A.S. had undisplaced fractures of the pubic bones. He was unable to void and complained of bladder pressure. Blood-tinged urine was removed by catheter. On intravenous urography, several loops of small bowel project into the opacified bladder. At operation, herniated small bowel was removed from the bladder and a posterior rupture was repaired.
(Courtesy of Stanford Rossiter, M.D., Sequoia Hospital, Redwood City, California.)

**FIGURE 13.8. DIAGRAM. RETRO-
PERITONEAL RUPTURE OF
THE BLADDER.**

Blood and urine infiltrate the retroperitoneal tissues at the base of the bladder.

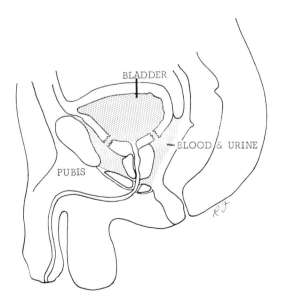

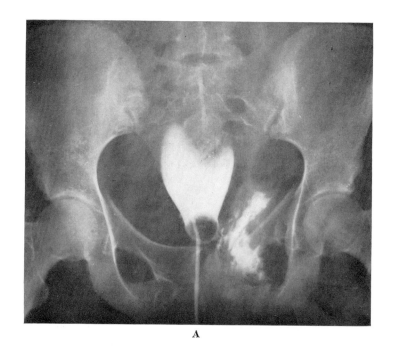

A

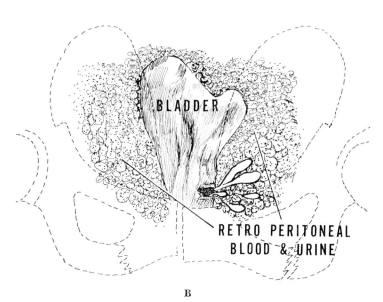

B

FIGURE 13.9. RETROPERITONEAL RUPTURE OF THE BLADDER.

A, Cystogram. G.T. had fractures of both pubic bones, with bilateral retroperitoneal hematomas. Cystography shows streaks of opaque medium in the retroperitoneal tissues. *B,* Diagram. This has a "sunburst" appearance characteristic of retroperitoneal extravasation.

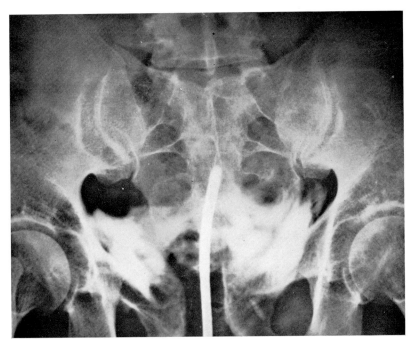

**FIGURE 13.10. RETROPERITONEAL RUPTURE OF THE BLADDER;
STREAK PATTERN.**

W.R. was admitted after a heavy timber had fallen across his abdomen. There
was separation of the symphysis pubis and sacroiliac joints. On cystography, the
opaque medium extends streak-like out into the retroperitoneal tissues. A ruptured bladder was found and repaired.

(Courtesy of George Hoeffler, M.D., Mills Memorial Hospital, San Mateo,
California.)

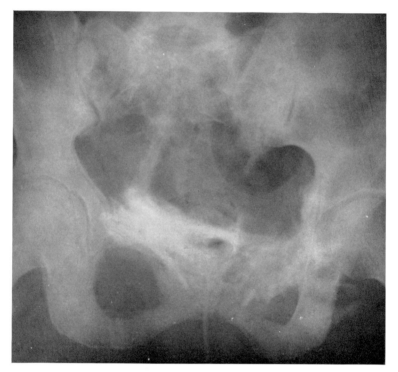

**FIGURE 13.11. RETROPERITONEAL RUPTURE OF THE BLADDER;
FRACTURE OF THE PUBIC BONES.**

M.R. after an automobile accident, the catheterized urine specimen was grossly
bloody. A cystogram shows a symmetrical position of the bladder with extensive
retroperitoneal extravasation. On continuous catheter drainage and antibiotics,
she made an uneventful recovery.

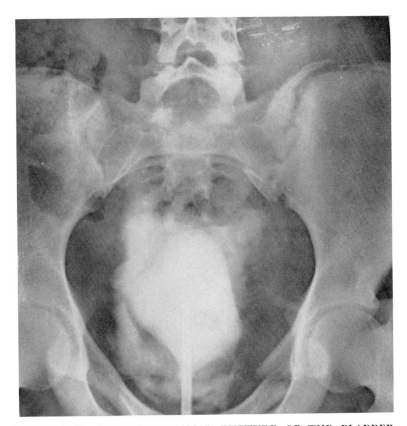

FIGURE 13.12. RETROPERITONEAL RUPTURE OF THE BLADDER.

L.P. had multiple pelvic fractures. The urine was grossly bloody. On cystography, the contrast medium extravasates into the retroperitoneal tissues. At operation, blood was found in the perivesical tissues due to two bladder lacerations. No intraperitoneal blood was found.

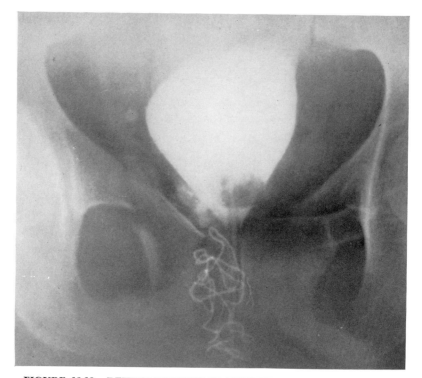

FIGURE 13.13. RETROPERITONEAL RUPTURE OF THE BLADDER.

L.M. had fractures of the inferior and superior rami of the pubic bones as well as vaginal laceration. This cystogram shows extravasation of the opaque medium into the retroperitoneal tissues on the right side. She made an uneventful recovery on conservative treatment.

REFERENCES

1. Bacon, S. K.: Rupture of the urinary bladder: Clinical analysis of 147 cases in the past ten years. J. Urol., *49*:432-435, 1943.
2. Beard, D. E., Goodyear, W. E., and Weens, H. S.: Radiologic Diagnosis of the Lower Urinary Tract. Springfield, Ill., Charles C Thomas, 1932, pp. 102-103.
3. Calhoon, H. W.: Trauma to bladder and posterior urethra. *In* Emmett, J. L.: Clinical Urography. An Atlas and Textbook of Roentgenologic Diagnosis. 2nd ed. Philadelphia, W. B. Saunders Co., 1964, pp. 1167-1179.
4. Edmondson, H. T., Jennings, W. D., and Rhode, C. M.: Pneumoperitoneum—A rare sign of urinary bladder rupture. Amer. Surg., *30*:721-724, 1964.
5. Kaiser, T. F., and Farrow, F. C.: Injury of the bladder and prostatomembranous urethra associated with fractures of the bony pelvis. Surg. Gynec. Obstet., *120*:99-112, 1965.
6. Lichtenheld, F. R., and Lancaster, J. M.: Intraperitoneal bladder rupture. J. Trauma, *2*:457-464, 1962.
7. Newland, D. E.: Genitourinary complications of pelvic fractures. J.A.M.A., *152*:1515-1520, 1953.
8. Prather, G. C.: Injuries of the bladder. Chapter 20 *in* Campbell, M. F. (ed.): Urology. 2nd ed. Philadelphia, W. B. Saunders Co., 1963.
9. Richardson, E. J.: Trauma to urethra and bladder in association with pelvic fractures. Minnesota Med., *34*:148-151, 1951.
10. Todd, I. A. D.: Genitourinary complications of blunt pelvic trauma. Canad. J. Surg., *7*:43, 1964.
11. Weens, H. S., Newman, J. H., and Florence, T. J.: Trauma of the lower urinary tract. A roentgenologic study. New Engl. J. Med., *234*:357-364, 1946.

14

LACERATION OF THE URETHRA

CLINICAL OBSERVATIONS

The patient with injury to the urethra is unable to void and there is gross bleeding from the urethra. If voiding is attempted, the patient has pain accompanied by increased swelling of the perineum or scrotum.[8] With severe trauma, the urethra may be avulsed from the bladder neck for a distance of several inches. Displacement of the urethra from the bladder is detected by digital examination of the rectum.[9, 10] Orkin[6] considers that this finding alone is sufficient for diagnosis and that further studies are unnecessary. Whenever it is impossible to pass a catheter through the urethra into the bladder, a separation of the urethra from the bladder is likely.[2]

ASSOCIATED INJURIES

Injury to the urethra above the urogenital diaphragm is most frequently associated with fracture of the pelvis, particularly of the pubic and ischial bones.[3, 10] A shearing force directed to the anterior pelvis pulls the bladder away from the urethra.

In the male, straddle injuries lead to rupture of the urethra below the urogenital diaphragm. Such injury is rare in the female. Fracture of the pelvis is not associated with straddle injury.

RADIOGRAPHIC EXAMINATION

Plain Film

Compression fractures of the pubis and ischium suggest the possibility of urethral laceration. Hemorrhage and extravasation in the pelvis will distort and obliterate the normal extraperitoneal fat and vesical outlines.

Urethrography

Twenty to 30 milliliters of 25 per cent sterile solution of a radiopaque contrast medium is injected through a Brodny urethral catheter. Films are obtained in the anteroposterior and both oblique projections. Extravasation at any point indicates urethral laceration.[7]

The cystographic study may be negative in the presence of urethral injury. Kaiser and Farrow[1] recommend that follow-up urethrography be done routinely in male patients with hematuria and negative cystograms.

TYPES OF URETHRAL INJURY

The radiographic changes depend on the relation of the urethral injury to the urogenital diaphragm. This diaphragm consists of two fascial layers which enclose the deep transverse peroneal muscle and the urogenital sphincter. Anteriorly, the two fascial layers are fused to form the transverse ligament of the pelvis. Posteriorly, the fascial layers are fused at the anal margin. The urethra, together with the blood and nerve supply to the penis (clitoris) penetrate both layers of fascia. In the female, the fascia is pierced by the vagina as well.[4] A barrier is formed by the urogenital diaphragm which limits and defines the extravasation of blood and urine in urethral injury.

Rupture above the Urogenital Diaphragm

With urethrography or cystography, the opaque medium passes into the perivesical retroperitoneal tissue (Figs. 14.1 and 14.2). The appearance is similar to that of the retroperitoneal rupture of the bladder. The extravasated opaque material fills the pelvis around the bladder base and has a "sunburst" appearance.

Rupture Below the Urogenital Diaphragm

Urethrography shows the passage of the opaque material into the perineum and scrotum (Figs. 14.3, 14.4 and 14.5). This is accompanied by increased swelling and induration of the perineal and scrotal tissues. Extravasated blood and urine in the perineum can lead to infection

(Text continued on page 226)

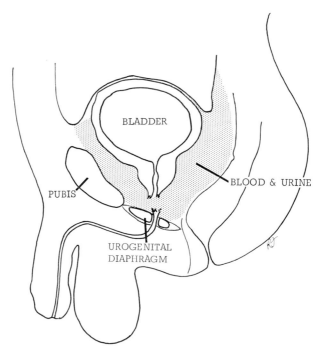

FIGURE 14.1.   DIAGRAM. RUPTURE OF THE URETHRA ABOVE THE UROGENITAL DIAPHRAGM.

Blood and urine infiltrate the retroperitoneal tissues.

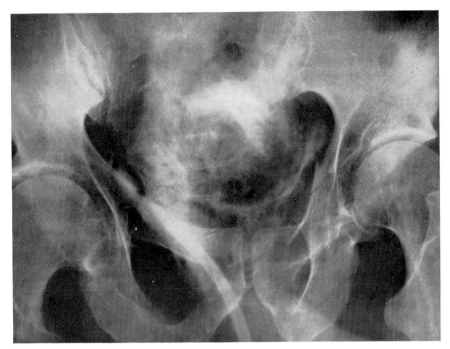

**FIGURE 14.2. RUPTURE OF THE URETHRA ABOVE THE UROGENITAL
DIAPHRAGM; RETROPERITONEAL EXTRAVASATION.**

E.D. sustained a severe crush fracture of the pelvis including the pubic bones
and ischia. On catheterization, blood was obtained. This cystourethrogram
shows opaque medium passing into the retroperitoneal tissues surrounding the
bladder. A rupture of the urethra just distal to the bladder orifice was found
and repaired.

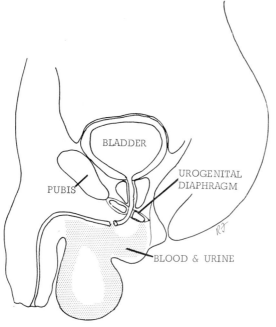

**FIGURE 14.3. DIAGRAM. LAC-
ERATION OF THE URETHRA
BELOW THE UROGENITAL
DIAPHRAGM.**

Blood and urine infiltrate the
perineum and scrotum.

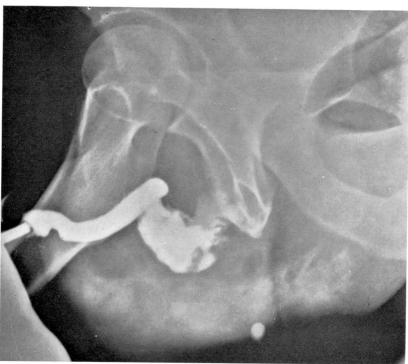

**FIGURE 14.4. RUPTURE OF THE URETHRA BELOW THE UROGENITAL
DIAPHRAGM; STRADDLE INJURY.**

C.C., a 34-year-old man, suffered a straddle injury. He had severe pain in the
groin and perineum and blood issued from the urethra. The physician was
unable to pass a small catheter. Urethrography shows a rupture of the caver-
nous urethra with extravasation into the scrotum.

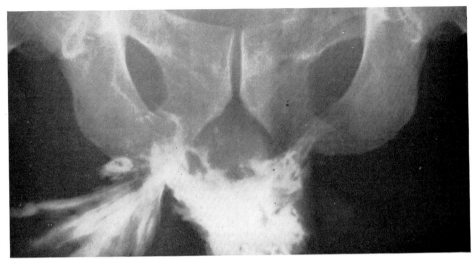

FIGURE 14.5. RUPTURE OF THE URETHRA BELOW THE UROGENITAL DIAPHRAGM; EXTRAVASATION INTO THE SCROTUM AND THIGH.

R.N. sustained a comminuted fracture of the left pubis and ischium. Grossly bloody urine was obtained on catheterization. Retrograde dye injection through a urethral catheter shows extravasation into the scrotum and right thigh.

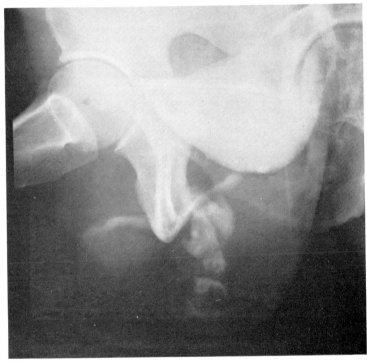

FIGURE 14.6. RUPTURE OF THE URETHRA BELOW THE UROGENITAL DIAPHRAGM; PERINEAL ABSCESS.

R.L. sustained a straddle injury. Five days later he developed a fluctuant area in the right perineal region. This was incised and there was profuse drainage of pus and urine. On urethrography there is extravasation into the perineum.

and abscess formation (Fig. 14.6). In very severe injuries to the pelvis, the urethra may rupture above and below the urogenital diaphragm, giving both types of bleeding and extravasation.

A complication of unrecognized or incompletely repaired urethral laceration is stricture formation.[1]

REFERENCES

1. Kaiser, T. F., and Farrow, F. C.: Injury of the bladder and prostatomembranous urethra associated with fracture of the bony pelvis. Surg. Gynec. Obstet., *120:* 99-112, 1965.
2. Lewis, L. G.: Traumatic injuries of the lower urinary tract. Amer. Surg., *23:* 1022-1029, 1957.
3. Lynch, K. M.: Traumatic urinary injuries. Pitfalls in their diagnosis and treatment. J. Urol. *77:*90-95, 1957.
4. Markee, J. E.: The urogenital system. *In* Schaeffer, J. P. (ed.): Morris' Human Anatomy. 11th ed. New York, Blakiston Division, McGraw-Hill Book Co., 1953, pp. 540-541.
5. Mulla, N., Storaci, F., and Lettiere, A. J.: Urethral injuries. Amer. J. Surg., *91:* 1004-1008, 1956.
6. Orkin, L. A.: Traumatic avulsion of bladder neck and prostate. Amer. J. Surg., *89:*840-853, 1953.
7. Ormond, J. K., and Fairey, P. W.: Urethral rupture at apex of prostate. Complication of fracture of pelvis. J.A.M.A., *149:*15-18, 1952.
8. Schulte, J. W.: Management of the severely injured patient—Genitourinary aspects. J.A.M.A., *168:*2094-2097, 1958.

15

RETROPERITONEAL HEMORRHAGE WITHOUT VISCERAL INJURY

CLINICAL OBSERVATIONS

Bleeding into the retroperitoneal tissues is not uncommon and is to be expected whenever there is injury to the muscles and bones which surround and support the abdomen. Ordinarily, this bleeding is not serious and is overshadowed by injury to the abdominal organs. At times, sizable hemorrhage can occur in the retroperitoneal soft tissues in the absence of visceral injury.

Clinical changes are: (1) a palpable mass in the pelvis or flank; (2) hypovolemic shock; (3) intestinal obstruction if the hematoma encroaches on the bowel lumen.

Retroperitoneal hemorrhages are usually self-limited and respond to conservative management.[3]

ASSOCIATED INJURIES

With fracture of the pelvis there is some degree of retroperitoneal bleeding, even in the absence of injury to the pelvic viscera. Braunstein et al.[2] studied 200 consecutive fatally injured pedestrians, 90 of whom had pelvic fractures. In 21 of the 90, retroperitoneal bleeding was signifi-cant; in 11, the fractured pelvis was the only source of a large hemorrhage found at autopsy. Baylis et al.[1] found that the retroperitoneal tissues may be the site of massive and unsuspected blood loss. Pelvic fractures with hemorrhage from the fracture site accounted for eight deaths in 127 fatal traffic accidents studied by Perry and McClellan.[5]

Because the leading cause of early death in pelvic fracture is massive hemorrhage, Hauser and Perry[4] recommend hypogastric artery ligation to control bleeding.

Retroperitoneal hemorrhage is also seen with fractures of the trans-verse processes of the lumbar spine and tears of the abdominal muscles.

RADIOGRAPHIC EXAMINATION

Plain Film

In the presence of fractures, particularly of the pelvis, asymmetry of the retroperitoneal fat lines is an indication of blood loss in the retro-peritoneal tissues.

Upper Gastrointestinal Series and Barium Enema

In the upper abdomen, retroperitoneal hematoma can encroach upon the lumen of the bowel where the peritoneum does not invest the intestine (bare area). Two common sites are periduodenal and retrocolic. The resultant narrowing of the bowel is shown by contrast study.

Intravenous Urogram and Cystogram

Within the bony pelvis, retroperitoneal hemorrhage displaces, com-presses or distorts the bladder. The degree of alteration of the bladder is an indication of the size of the hematoma.

TYPES OF RETROPERITONEAL HEMORRHAGE

Radiographically, retroperitoneal hemorrhage is seen in four areas of the abdomen: (1) pelvic, (2) periduodenal, (3) retrocolic and (4) para-vertebral.

Pelvic

Pelvic retroperitoneal hemorrhage is recognized by displacement of the peritoneal fat, the bladder or the rectum (Fig. 15.1).

(Text continued on page 232)

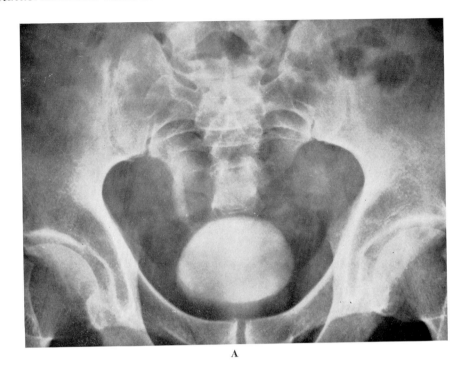

A

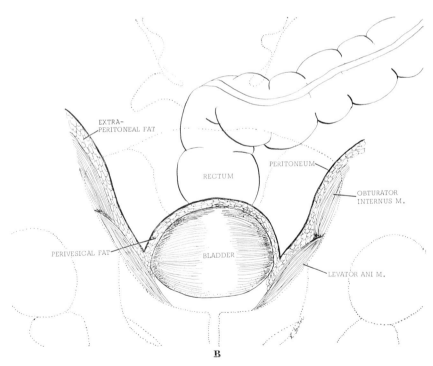

B

FIGURE 15.1. EXTRAPERITONEAL FAT LINES OF THE PELVIS.

A, Normal pelvis. The inner wall of the bladder is shown by diatrizoate and the outer wall by perivesical fat. *B*, Diagram. Laterally the extraperitoneal fat outlines the obturator internus muscle and inferiorly it outlines the levator ani muscle. The rectum is seen when it contains gas and stool.

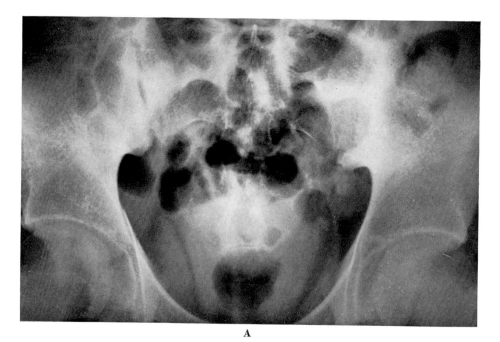

A

B

FIGURE 15.2. RETROPERITONEAL HEMORRHAGE; MEDIAL DISPLACEMENT OF THE EXTRAPERITONEAL FAT LINE.

A, AP film. W.D. suffered a fracture of the right acetabulum. A hematoma surrounds the fracture and displaces the extraperitoneal fat line medially. *B,* Diagram.

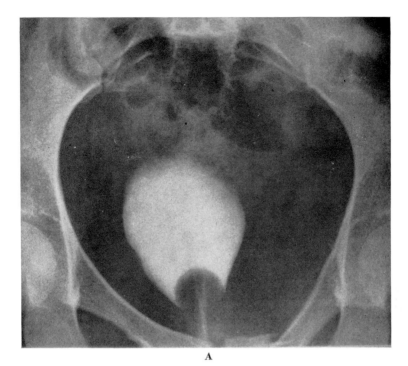

A

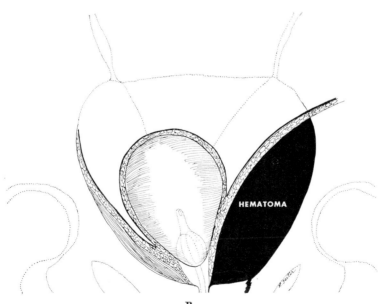

HEMATOMA

B

**FIGURE 15.3. PELVIC RETROPERITONEAL HEMORRHAGE; COMPRESSION AND
UPWARD DISPLACEMENT OF THE BLADDER ("TEAR-DROP BLADDER").**

A, Cystogram. J.C., a 19-year-old girl had been thrown to the pavement in an
automobile accident. *B,* Diagram. There is a fracture of the left pubic bone,
and a large retroperitoneal hematoma elevates and compresses the dye-filled
urinary bladder.

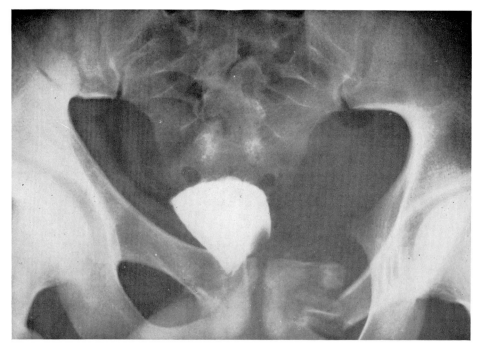

**FIGURE 15.4. PELVIC RETROPERITONEAL HEMORRHAGE; "TEAR-DROP BLADDER";
MUCOSAL LACERATION.**

M.A. had a severely comminuted fracture of both pubic bones and the right
ilium. After intravenous urography, the bladder is found deviated to the right
side by a large retroperitoneal hematoma. The slight irregularity of the left
side of the bladder indicates an associated mucosal tear.

With small hemorrhage, the pelvic peritoneal fat line, adjacent to
the fracture, is displaced toward the midline (Fig. 15.2).

With anterior extension of the hemorrhage, the bladder is compressed
and elongated, "the tear-drop bladder" (Figs. 15.3 and 15.4).[6] Hemorrhage
also elevates the bladder above the pelvic floor. This is best demonstrated
by opacifying the bladder.

When the hemorrhage extends posteriorly, the rectum is displaced
from the midline (Fig. 15.5). An air enema is used to outline the rectum
and sigmoid if displacement is suspected.

Periduodenal

Following injury, a hematoma can form in the periduodenal retroperitoneal tissues without a discoverable tear in the wall of the intestine. As
the hematoma enlarges, it encroaches on the lumen of the duodenum in
a manner similar to that of intramural bleeding (Chapter 9). Within a
short time after the accident, persistent vomiting develops. On the upper
gastrointestinal study, the retroperitoneal portion of the duodenum is

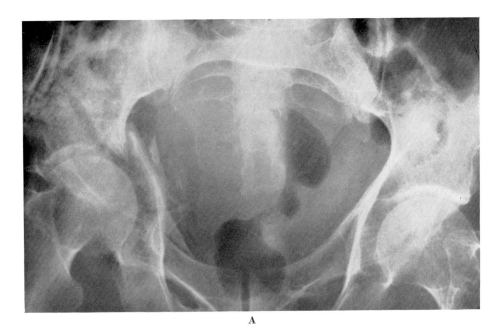

A

PERITONEUM

HEMATOMA

FRACTURE

RECTUM

B

**FIGURE 15.5. PELVIC RETROPERITONEAL HEMORRHAGE; COMPRESSION
AND DISPLACEMENT OF THE RECTUM.**

A, AP film. R.K. sustained a severely comminuted fracture of the innominate
bone. A large hematoma in the right retroperitoneal soft tissues of the pelvis
displaces the rectosigmoid colon to the opposite side. *B,* Diagram. Follow-up
films showed healing of the fracture, absorption of the hematoma, and a return
of the rectum to the midline.

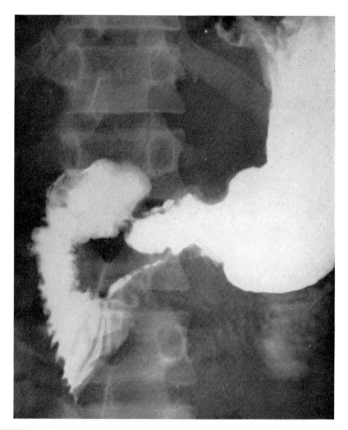

FIGURE 15.6. PERIDUODENAL HEMORRHAGE WITH OBSTRUCTION.

Twenty-four hours after striking his abdomen against the steering wheel, D.H. developed abdominal cramps with vomiting. An obstruction to the third portion of the duodenum is present. At operation, there was a retroperitoneal hematoma compressing the third portion of the duodenum. The peritoneal and retroperitoneal organs were intact.

(Courtesy of T. Hattori, M.D., Monterey, California.)

compressed, with flattening and effacement of the valvulae conniventes (Fig. 15.6).

Relief of obstruction is obtained by evacuating the hematoma.

Retrocolic

Retroperitoneal hemorrhage in the bare area behind the colon compresses the lumen of the bowel. Radiographically, it resembles intramural hemorrhage. The haustra of the colon are flattened and the space between them is widened (Figs. 15.7 and 15.8).

(Text continued on page 239)

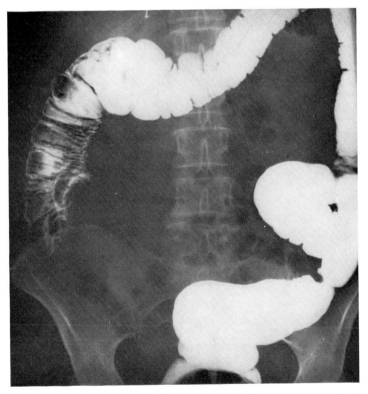

**FIGURE 15.7. RETROCOLIC HEMORRHAGE COMPRESSING AND
NARROWING THE CECUM.**

C.S. had generalized clonic convulsions. A mass is seen pressing on the posteromedial margin of the cecum with flattening of the mucosal markings. At operation, the mass was a discrete encapsulated hematoma with no visceral injury. The hemorrhage is thought to have resulted from soft tissue injury during the patient's convulsions.

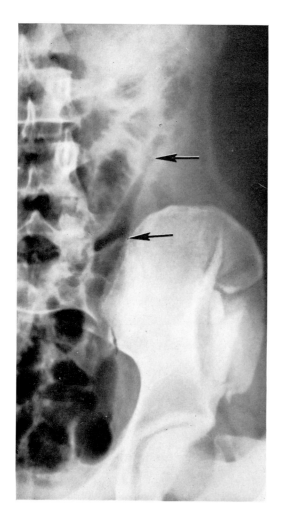

**FIGURE 15.8. RETROCOLIC HEM-
ORRHAGE; COMPRESSION OF
THE DESCENDING COLON;
FRACTURE OF THE ILIUM.**

D.H. suffered a severely comminuted fracture of the left
ilium, with several indriven
fragments. This radiograph
shows a large hematoma above
the fracture between the extraperitoneal fat and the colon.
The descending colon is displaced medially and is compressed by the hematoma (arrows). Follow-up films showed
absorption of the hematoma.

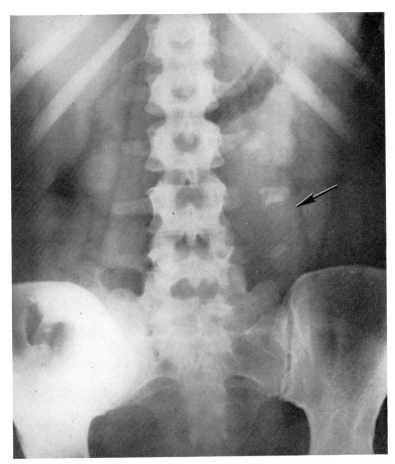

**FIGURE 15.9. RETROPERITONEAL PARAVERTEBRAL HEMORRHAGE;
FRACTURE OF THE TRANSVERSE PROCESS.**

M.I. had fractures of the left transverse processes of L3, L4 and L5. The lower pole of the left kidney is obscured. The extraperitoneal fat, which outlines the psoas muscle, is irregular and is displaced laterally (arrow). At operation, a large hemorrhage surrounded the left psoas muscle and had reflected the descending colon medially.

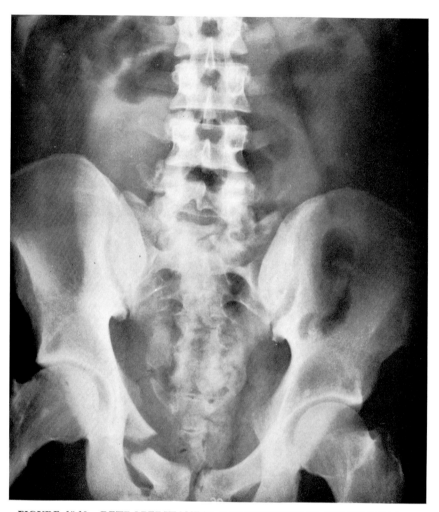

**FIGURE 15.10. RETROPERITONEAL PARAVERTEBRAL HEMORRHAGE;
CONTUSION OF THE RIGHT PSOAS MUSCLE.**

J.B. The psoas muscle outlines are asymmetrical because of a bulge on the right.
The extraperitoneal fat over the psoas is displaced laterally. Comminuted
fractures of the left transverse process of L5, the right sacrum and right pubic
bones are present. At operation, a large hematoma surrounding the right psoas
muscle was evacuated.

Paravertebral

Hemorrhage into the paravertebral soft tissues accompanies fractures of the transverse processes of the lumbar vertebrae or injury to the psoas muscle. As a result, the muscle outline is widened and irregular. The layer of fat which covers the muscle is displaced laterally (Figs. 15.9 and 15.10).

REFERENCES

1. Baylis, S. M., Lansing, E. H., and Glas, W. W.: Traumatic retroperitoneal hematoma. Amer. J. Surg., *103:*477-480, 1962.
2. Braunstein, P. W., Skudder, P. A., McCarroll, J. R., Masolino, A., and Wade, P. A.: Concealed hemorrhage due to pelvic fracture. J. Trauma, *4:*832-838, 1964.
3. Cushman, G. F.: Subperitoneal hemorrhage. Calif. Med., *78:*11-16, 1953.
4. Hauser, C. W., and Perry, J. F.: Control of massive hemorrhage from pelvic fractures by hypogastric artery ligation. Surg. Gynec. Obstet., *121:*313-315, 1965.
5. Perry, J. F., and McClellan, R. J.: Autopsy findings in 127 patients following fatal traffic accidents. Surg. Gynec. Obstet., *119:*586-590, 1964.
6. Prather, A. G., and Kaiser, T. F.: The bladder in fracture of the bony pelvis. The significance of a "tear drop" bladder as shown on a cystogram. J. Urol., *13:*1019, 1950.

16

INFREQUENT ABDOMINAL INJURIES

LACERATIONS OF UTERUS, TUBES OR OVARIES

Clinical Observations

Laceration of the uterus, tubes or ovaries is rare and has no characteristic radiographic signs. With mild trauma, a hematoma develops in the involved organs. With severe trauma and vessel laceration, there may be free bleeding into the peritoneal cavity. This is recognized by the signs of blood in the flanks and pelvis. Bleeding from the reproductive organs is not profuse and these injuries are rarely fatal.[8]

Injury to the Gravid Uterus

When gravid, the uterus is more susceptible to injury, particularly in the last trimester. In this period, a tear or rupture of the uterus results in death of the fetus and massive intra-abdominal hemorrhage.[4, 11] Because of profound blood loss and serious injury to the uterus, hysterectomy is frequently necessary.

Radiographically, the continuity of the uterine outline is lost and fluid is present in the flanks. A position of the fetus high in the abdomen or a posture which shows no adjustment to the surrounding uterine muscle suggests uterine rupture.[5, 12]

240

Injury to the Fetus

Fetal death can occur without damage to the uterine wall and cases have been described in which the fetal skeleton or skull has been fractured inside the intact uterus.[1, 3, 6, 7, 10] In one case, death was attributed to a fragment of the maternal pubic bone driven into the fetal skull.[9] In approximately one half of the reported cases, fetal death resulted from premature separation of the placenta.[2]

VASCULAR INJURY

Aorta and Iliac Arteries

Major injury to the abdominal aorta is usually fatal and the patient does not reach the emergency room for definitive care. Traumatic aneurysm of the abdominal aorta is rare.

A complication of iliac artery contusion is intravascular thrombosis.[14, 15] Clinically, the leg supplied by the artery is pulseless and cold and there are signs of impending gangrene (Fig. 16.1). The degree and extent of arterial injury is determined by arteriography.[15] Morris, Creech and DeBakey[18] report on seven iliac artery injuries that were treated surgically. The pulses were restored in four instances. Immediate repair by anastomosis or homograft replacement is recommended.

Injuries of the major branches of the abdominal aorta are rarely reported. Stutz et al.[22] describe a patient with post-traumatic aneurysm of the gastroduodenal artery. Ulvestad[23] found a traumatic laceration of the superior mesenteric artery in one patient.

Trauma to the abdomen is reported to cause thrombosis of the hepatic artery.[13, 16]

Inferior Vena Cava and Pelvic Veins

Injury to the inferior vena cava and pelvic veins is accompanied by massive blood loss (Fig. 16.2). This injury has a very high mortality.[17, 19] In three patients with vena cava injury reported by Schuck and Trump,[21] death occurred before the defect in the vessel could be repaired.

Traumatic occlusion of the hepatic vein results in liver failure and ascites (the Budd-Chiari syndrome).[20]

Cysterna Chyli

An unusual instance of chylous peritonitis with pseudocyst has been recorded as a complication of blunt trauma.[24]

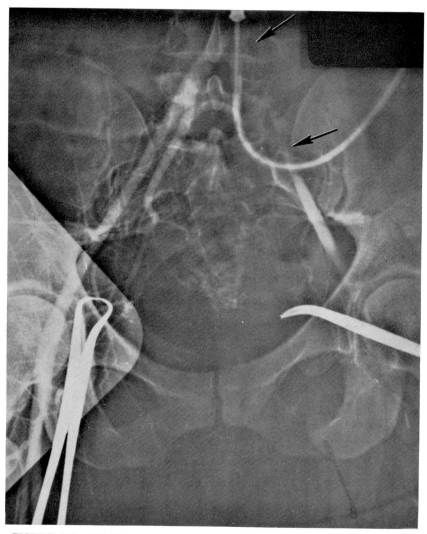

**FIGURE 16.1.   TRAUMATIC OCCLUSION OF THE LEFT ILIAC ARTERY;
OPERATIVE ARTERIOGRAM.**

L.F. had pulseless left leg following abdominal contusion. At abdominal exploration, the left common iliac artery was found to have been avulsed from the aorta,
with only remnants of the adventitia intact. Distally, the lumen was occluded by
the retraction of the intima and media. After injection of diatrizoate sodium
into the aorta, there is no filling of the left iliac (between arrows). Subsequent
injection into the left common femoral artery showed the vessels patent below
the occlusion. The injured segment was replaced by a Teflon graft.
(Courtesy of Robert Allansmith, M.D., San Jose, California.)

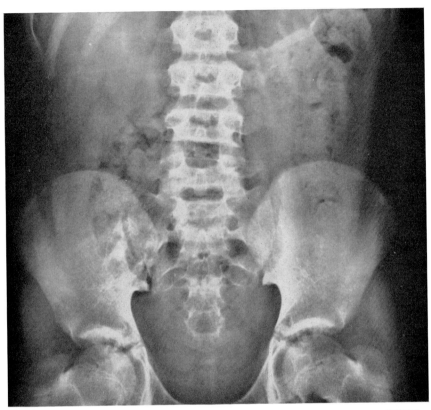

**FIGURE 16.2. LACERATIONS OF THE INFERIOR VENA CAVA AND LIVER;
MASSIVE HEMOPERITONEUM.**

B.S. After a piece of heavy equipment had fallen on his abdomen, he was in
shock with hematocrit of 30 and blood pressure 80/50. There is blood in the
peritoneum between the colon and the fat line bilaterally and in the pelvic
recesses. Operation was performed immediately. The copious amount of blood
came from an open laceration of the vena cava and a fracture of the right lobe
of the liver.
(Courtesy of George Hoeffler, M.D., Mills Memorial Hospital, San Mateo,
California.)

REFERENCES

Trauma to Uterus, Tubes and Ovaries

1. Broadbent, T. R., and Hochstrasser, A.: Fracture of the mandibular condyle in the newborn. Plast. Reconstr. Surg., 20:171-175, 1957.
2. Dyer, I., and Barclay, D. L.: Accidental trauma complicating pregnancy and delivery. Am. J. Obstet. Gynec., 21:477-480, 1963.
3. Jones, G. F., and O'Nan, W. L.: Intrauterine skull fracture. Kentucky Med. J., 38:273, 1940.
4. McClure, J. N., Jr.: Rupture of the pregnant uterus due to non-penetrating abdominal trauma. Surgery, 35:487-490, 1954.
5. Parkinson, C. E.: Traumatic rupture of the gravid uterus. Amer. J. Roentgenol., 80:684-685, 1958.
6. Parkinson, E. B.: Perinatal loss due to external trauma to the uterus. Amer. J. Obstet. Gynec., 90:30-33, 1964.
7. Pike, J. B.: In utero depressed fracture of fetal skull. Med. Times, 86:869-871, 1958.
8. Quast, D. C., and Jordan, G. L.: Traumatic wounds of the female reproductive organs. J. Trauma, 4:839-844, 1964.
9. Seear, T., and Woeppel, C. J.: Traumatic fetal death resulting from fractured pelvis. Amer. J. Obstet. Gynec., 83:907-926, 1962.
10. Theurer, D. E., and Kaiser, I. H.: Traumatic fetal death without uterine injury. Report of a case. Obstet. Gynec., 21:477-480, 1963.
11. Ulvestad, L. E.: Repair of laceration of superior mesenteric artery acquired by nonpenetrating injury to abdomen. Ann. Surg., 140:752-755, 1954.
12. Wondrok, E., and Minarikova, E.: Die chylose Peritonitis und chylose Pseudozyste als seltene Spotefolge eines steumpfen Bauchtrauma. Zentralbl. Chir., 86: 1130-1134, 1961.

Vascular Injury

13. Brink, A. J., and Botha, D.: Budd-Chiari syndrome. Diagnosis by hepatic venography. Brit. J. Radiol., 28:330-331, 1955.
14. Collins, H. A., and Jacobs, J. K.: Acute arterial injuries due to blunt trauma. J. Bone & Joint Surg., 43A:193-197, 1961.
15. Couves, C. M., Lumpkin, M. B., and Howard, J. M.: Arterial injuries due to blunt (non-penetrating) trauma. Experiences with fifteen patients. Canad. J. Surg., 1:197-200, 1958.
16. Little, R. D., and Montgomery, P. O'B.: Case report of stenosis of the vena cava with vena caval and hepatic vein thrombosis related to trauma. Ann. Int. Med., 37:197-203, 1952.
17. Martin, J. D., Perdue, G. D., and Harrison, W. H.: Abdominal injury due to nonpenetrating trauma. A.M.A. Arch. Surg., 80:192-197, 1960.
18. Morris, G. C., Creech, O., Jr., and DeBakey, M. E.: Acute Arterial Injuries in Civilian Practice. Amer. J. Surg., 93:565-572, 1957.
19. Ochsner, J. L., Crawford, E. S., and DeBakey, M. E.: Injuries of the vena cava caused by external trauma. Surgery, 49:397-405, 1961.
20. Parker, R. G. F.: Occlusion of the hepatic veins in man. Medicine, 38:369-392, 1959.
21. Schuck, J. M., and Trump, D. S.: Nonpenetrating abdominal trauma with injury to blood vessels. Amer. Surgeon, 21:693-697, 1961.
22. Stulz, E., Naett, R., and Anger, R.: Reflexions à propos d'un cas d'aneurysme de rupture de l'artere gastro-duodenale consecutif à un traumatisme ferme de l'abdomen. Lyon Chir., 57:440-443, 1961.
23. Woodhull, R. B.: Traumatic rupture of the pregnant uterus resulting from an automobile accident. Surgery, 12:615, 1942.
24. Zuppinger, A.: Roentgen diagnostics in obstetrics. In Schinz, H. R., Baensch, W. E., Friedl, E., and Uehlinger, E.: Roentgen-Diagnostics. New York, Grune and Stratton, 1954.

Index

Page numbers in *italics* indicate illustrations.

245